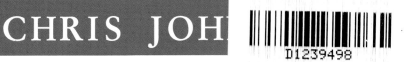

CHRIS JOH

MEAL PATTERNING

DEVELOPING HEALTHY NUTRITIONAL PATTERNS FOR A LIFETIME

ISBN 0-9727281-0-4

First Printing 2003

Printed in the United States of America

Design by:
Ciesa & Associates
East Lansing, MI

Photos by: Tom Gennera and Ciesa & Associates

Cover Design: Ciesa & Associates

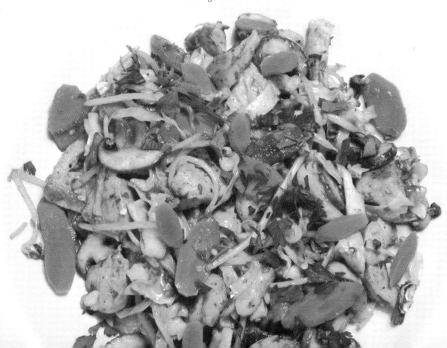

Table of Contents

Section I
Meal Patterning Is a Way of Life

Section 2
Steps to Success

Section 3
Tools for Success—A Guide to Everyday Life

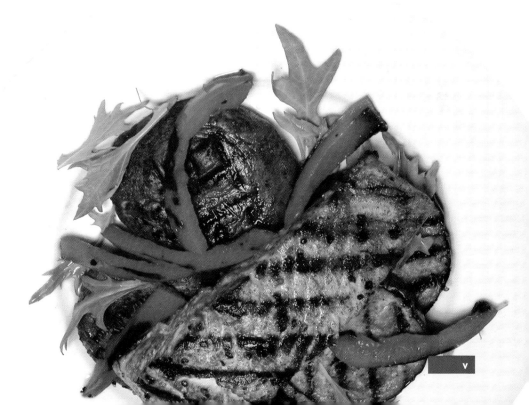

Acknowledgements / Dedication

There are so many people who were instrumental in the development and completion of this book. I'd like to begin by thanking a few of my college professors, Dr. Louis Junker, Dr. Wayne Van Huss, Dr. William Heusner and Dr. Kwok Ho for sharing their passion and opening my eyes to a career in the health and fitness industry. To JoAnn James and my good friend and colleague Dan Bender for making graduate school a very enjoyable experience.

To Lisa Crumley whose prodding, pushing and patience played a large role in writing this book.

To many of my personal training clients who have edited, supported and inspired this project every step of the way, Dr. Janet Osuch, Jill Dehlin, Jerry King, Carol Conn, Dr. Carol Levin, Lev Rapheal, Gersh Kaufman, Dr. Ralph Harvey, Bob Cornwell, Dr. Teresa Bernardez, Mary Beth Scheffel, Ann Shneider, Pam Flewelling, Michele Meyrowitz and Dr. Cynthia Hockett.

To Michelle Nikoli, R.D. for her professional approach and expertise in the editing of this book.

To Steve Trego and Diane Layman at Ideas at Work for all your hard work and patience in putting this book together.

To Carl Porter and Mike Combes for your support and standing behind this project from the very beginning.

To Lauren Ciesa, Peter Lusch, Ben Gaydos and Gerna Rubenstein for your guidance, creativity and vision in bringing this project to completion.

To Waymer Moore, my exercise model, for your warm smile.

To Ingrid Hinde for spreading the Meal Patterning message all over the world. Your energy, passion and perseverance are infectious with everyone you meet.

To Al Arens, for your advice, guidance and friendship which were so helpful in keeping me on the right path.

To Mary Kishler for your two cents. Hugs and smiles!

To my buddy Ed Thorpe, for your positive outlook on life and kindness.

To the team of personal trainers thanks for your warmth, passion and spirit, you make coming to work a real joy.

To my Thursday afternoon foursome — John, Dennie, Rick and Berger — I love you all like brothers.

To my mom, dad, sister and brother for your love and support. You encouraged me to chase my dreams.

And finally, to my wife, Paula, and my kids, Kristen and Matt, for giving me the time, support and all your love.

Thanks.
CJ

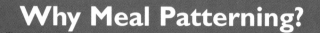

Why Meal Patterning?

Let food be your medicine and medicine be your food.
– Hippocrates

As director of fitness and co-director of personal training at one of the largest hospital-based health clubs in the world, I have the privilege of helping people improve the quality of their lives through changes in lifestyle, especially exercise and nutrition. It is rewarding to help people begin nutritional changes that they slowly adopt, adapt to, live with and then enjoy.

One of my greatest challenges, whether working one-on-one with a client, instructing new personal trainers or speaking to large audiences, is making nutritional information easy to understand.

I developed the concept of Meal Patterning about ten years ago. I watched and listened as people tried any and every weight loss program that hit the bestseller list. Sooner or later, most would come back to their original nutritional patterns—their own meal patterns. They were not educated about nutrition. They just followed the newest diet or plan with the hope of developing the bodies of their dreams.

> **I believe most people have three goals when it comes to their nutritional programs.**
>
> 1. **To control their weight.** Whether it's to maintain, decrease or even increase body weight, they want to be in control of their own bodies.
> 2. **To feel good and have energy throughout the day.**
> 3. **To maintain or improve their health.**
>
> **With Meal Patterning you can achieve all three.**

We are obsessed with weight loss in the United States, spending $50 billion per year in the weight loss industry. Yet we are still a nation that is overweight and physically limited.

Meal Patterning begins by laying the foundation of nutritional education. I will explain why obesity in the United States is climbing so quickly. Why diets don't work. How to understand the function of the three macronutrients—carbohydrates, proteins and fats. How carbohydrates impact your energy, waistline and mood. How proteins help control food cravings, improve brainpower and increase energy. How certain fats are essential for long-term health and weight control, while other fats lead to disease and make you fat. I will give you the nutritional knowledge that will allow you to make informed, good, healthy and empowering decisions related to the food you eat.

The second half of Meal Patterning is about changing nutritional patterns. People are challenged by change, especially when it comes to the food they eat. I will show you how to make small changes to your current nutritional patterns that you can maintain for your lifetime. You will look at food in a completely different way.

I have also included a section on exercise and staying motivated and empowered. Learn what Meal Patterning can do for you. Get on board—come take the Meal Patterning ride with me and all the others who love this way of eating and living. You're worth it.

— C.J.

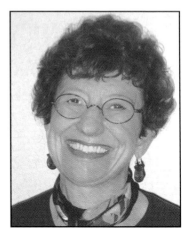

" Having been one of those uncoordinated kids in school, hating PE and always picked last for any mandatory school team, I found all kinds of excuses not to exercise as an adult. I didn't like it, it was for people who cared about having a super attractive body to attract a mate, I didn't have time. You name it–I had an excuse. As a physician, I knew that this wasn't very wise, but also rationalized that my estrogen would protect me from the ravages of heart disease.

And eating! Well, I thought I was eating pretty well, when I did eat, which wasn't regularly. A typical menu? Coffee for breakfast. Lunch? Not having time to prepare a lunch before tearing out the door at 6:30 AM to begin my day, having few places to buy a decent lunch near my work, and being pressured to "work in" patients over the noon hour meant that I often ate lunch only when a colleague or I scheduled it over a work issue, or when I was so hungry I felt like I would faint if I didn't get something in my body soon. Typically, that might mean a candy bar. Ironically enough, during this time I counseled patients on the importance of a healthy lifestyle, including regular eating and exercising. But oh, I had a large low-fat meal consisting of lots of fruits and vegetables at night, to be sure! And I avoided fast-food restaurants as much as possible. How much more healthy can you get?

My wake-up call for a lifestyle change came on February 27, 1998, when I was diagnosed with a benign brain tumor that was large enough to be causing symptoms requiring neurosurgical intervention. When I awoke from the post-operative coma 10 days later, I weighed less than 100 pounds. What little muscle I had had almost disappeared, and I couldn't walk. In fact, I couldn't even sit up straight in my wheelchair. My rehabilitation consisted of 6 hours a day, 5 days a week of intensive therapy for a month, followed by 8-10 hours per week of therapy over the next year. At the end of it, my physical rehabilitation therapist met with my new personal trainer, Chris Johnson, to help me transition between formal rehabilitation and personal training for one hour per week.

To my surprise, the first month that Chris and I met consisted mostly of nutritional counseling. I learned about all the eating mistakes that I was making and how to adapt eating habits that were to become life-long. The exercise regimen that he helped me establish has helped me understand that you don't need to be a professional athlete to care about your body and to help it function at an optimal level. The healthy lifestyle that I now lead has contributed enormously to my emotional well-being as well.

The contribution of Chris's mentoring, guidance and caring has had a profound impact on my life. The circumstances of my need for his message are ones that I would not wish for any of you. I do, however, wish for each of you to be receptive to his message. It truly can change your life. It certainly changed mine. **"**

—Janet Rose Osuch, MD

Section 1

Meal Patterning is a Way of Life

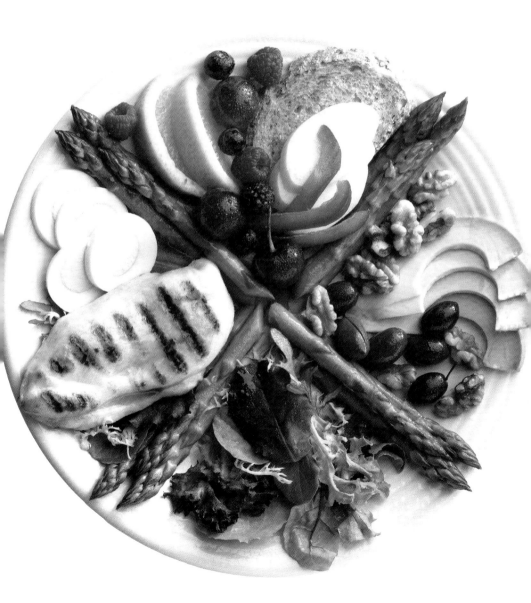

Chapter 1

Meal Patterning is a Way of Life–It's Not a Diet

Prevention is so much better than healing.
— Thomas Adams

Meal Patterning is learning to nourish your body so that you function at your optimum level. Think of this book as your chance to start over with a fresh approach to food and nutrition. It is your opportunity to debunk outdated theories about eating. Meal Patterning opens the door to understanding how the food you eat affects not just your weight or your long-term health, but your feeling of well-being and performance in every aspect of your life. Following simple Meal Patterning principles, you open the door to optimal health and peak performance, both for your body and your life. Meal Patterning is a powerful tool that is readily available to you, right here, right now.

Think about it. Most diet programs don't work for many reasons. A fundamental flaw of dieting is the "prescription" approach. The diet is like a prescription: follow a very specific, prescribed plan for a specific, prescribed period of time to achieve a specific, prescribed result. Dieters are directed to simply follow the prescribed plan with neither an explanation of the nutritional science behind it, nor an understanding of how or why the program works, nor what other lifestyle changes are required to enjoy a lifelong improvement in health. Without knowledge, dieters are powerless over situations that don't exactly follow the prescription. Dieters lack options because they lack the knowledge to make healthy, reasonable choices. Once they stop "taking their prescription," they lose the benefit, or intended result. Worst of all, perhaps, in the diet scenario is the single focus on losing weight, without paying the necessary attention to overall health and well-being.

> 66 What a delight to hear someone speak in such a positive way about diet. The first three letters of that word make most people discouraged after any interval of trying to make it work. Your presentation was one of the better ones that I have seen.
>
> The patients who I see are what I call the "walking wounded." Using those principals that you shared during your conference and helping them to reduce the reactions that they have to their environment, they slowly become the "walking delighted. 99
>
> – Douglas F. Wacker, MD, FAAO-HNS, FACS, FAAOA

You don't have to be like dieters. When you begin to learn the basics of good nutrition through Meal Patterning, your options will be unlimited. You will have the knowledge and the tools you need to make smart, healthy choices whether you are at the grocery store, a restaurant, a party or in your own kitchen tweaking your favorite recipe. Some of my most rewarding moments as a personal trainer are when I hear clients report that they successfully handled a challenging situation with food, and when I see their sense of pride and accomplishment, knowing they have not let themselves down. Many say it wasn't nearly as hard as they thought it would be because they were armed with the right information. That's the point of Meal Patterning—to arm you with the right information so you can make healthy, self-enhancing, empowering nutritional choices for yourself, and to develop Meal Patterning habits that will stay with you for a lifetime.

Sort Information from Misinformation

Many of my clients are frustrated with the overwhelming amount of nutrition information available. Studies release conflicting data every day. There's so much information that people find it difficult to keep up with it all and to sort out what is legitimate from what isn't. In the following chapters, I will synthesize information from hundreds of competent, reliable sources and make it easy to understand.

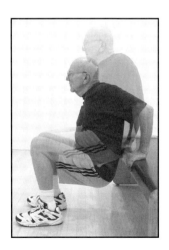

66 Meal Patterning has had a positive influence on my life. I've lost 35 pounds and moved from 24 to 15 percent body fat. More importantly, this healthy weight has held steady for three years by applying the Meal Patterning strategy and exercise.

Meal Patterning empowers me to make "right" choices about eating—what, when and how much. The goal is to stop storage of fat rather than trying to control appetite. My quality of life in general has improved because of Meal Patterning. 99

**– Roger Niemeyer,
Professor of Education**

Optimize Your Health

Nutrition is the foundation of good health. Creating optimal health includes several factors, but it begins with nutrition.

As your life becomes more complex, it is important to focus on the basics. Strive to create balance in your life. The key to success and enjoyment in life is finding balance in the goals you set nutritionally, physically, socially, professionally and spiritually.

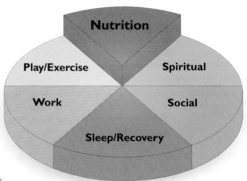

I am amazed that people often take better care of their pets and plants—even their houses and automobiles—than they do their own bodies. People protect their investment in their cars by performing routine maintenance and using the proper fuel and motor oil. Your body is the only one you will ever have. Invest in yourself and protect your investment.

The Diet Roller Coaster– Why Diets Don't Work

Why are we trying harder to lose weight and failing more than ever? There are four primary reasons: poor information; a decline in the quality of food most readily available; a pervasive dieting mentality; and, lack of exercise.

1. **Poor information:** Diets advocated through popular culture, the media and the outdated food pyramid leave food consumers in a state of flux and confusion.

2. **Decline in the quality of food:** We are a nation of convenience-food consumers. Convenience translates into highly processed, poor-quality food. As the speed of our lives increases, so does the demand for convenient, fast, available food. Food companies sell us poor-quality food because we continue to buy it. Until we begin to change our buying practices,

manufacturers will continue to produce poor-quality, nutritionally-deficient foods. As consumers become more educated about eating quality foods, demand for quality foods will grow.

3. **Pervasive dieting mentality:** Over the last 30 years, a plethora of fad diets and trendy ways of eating has bombarded Americans. New books, magazines, testimonials and infomercials bring the promise of instant weight loss and fitness. With each promise, it's easy to see why many of us will try any new diet that comes along if the claims are powerful enough.

4. **Lack of exercise:** As our lives speed up, the time we spend being physically active continues to decline. Our kids seldom walk to school. They sit in the classroom, sit behind the computer after school and sit watching television. Less than 30 percent of U.S. adults exercise regularly. Regular exercise has many wonderful benefits, but many choose not to make time for regular exercise.

> **❝** Your Meal Patterning program has saved my life and changed me tremendously.
>
> I have now a much healthier relationship with food and can live with this program for the rest of my life. I feel and look so much better. I weighed 338 pounds just two years ago. I am down to 180 as of today, so have now lost 158 pounds and am still losing. Granted, it's been a long road and a lot of hard work– but the result is more than worth it.
>
> The weight I have lost is only half as important as what I have gained: self-confidence; incredible pride and a belief in myself; the satisfaction of knowing I have done the impossible; the respect and admiration of other people; the joy of finally being able to experience life; and, the incredible health benefits that come from finally having the right tool to lead a healthy and productive life. Chris Johnson's Meal Patterning is a plan that I can easily – and very happily – live with for the rest of my life. **❞**
>
> – **Ingrid L. Hinde,**
>   **Fairbanks, AK**

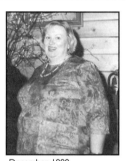

December 1999
338 lbs. (size 28)

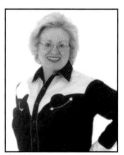

April 2003
190 lbs. (size 14/16)

Chapter 2

The Simple Truth About Diets

Our life is what our thoughts make it.
— Marcus Aurelius

Hundreds of new diet programs hit the market every year. The American population is obsessed with weight loss and is always searching for new and better ways to lose weight. Without understanding some of the basic principles for successful weight loss, dieters will continue to search for the magic plan that is "right" for them. Let's examine some of the diets that capture people's attention with promises of quick, painless weight loss.

Scenario 1

Low-Fat, Low-Protein, High-Carbohydrate Diet

Most consumers know that one gram of fat produces nine calories; more than twice that of carbohydrate and protein. In this diet, fat is the villain. This diet drastically reduces or eliminates dietary fat and replaces it with low-fat/no-fat products. It also severely restricts meat to control dietary fat. Here is a typical day in the life of this dieter.

Breakfast	bagel cream cheese orange juice coffee
Snack	apple

Lunch	salad with vegetables
	fat-free raspberry
	  vinaigrette dressing
	1 piece whole grain
	  bread

Snack	2 rice cakes 2 pieces of hard candy

Dinner	pasta with Marinara
	  sauce
	salad with non-fat
	  dressing
	2 bread sticks

Snack	air-popped popcorn

The diet allows water, coffee and diet soda freely throughout the day and with meals. It discourages most snacking, though it allows some light snacking on vegetables.

Nutritionally, the composition of this diet is grossly unbalanced and depends heavily on carbohydrates as the primary source of calories at every meal. The intent of the diet is to restrict calories by reducing dietary fat in the hope that there will be a corresponding reduction in body fat.

The first problem is that restriction of dietary fat doesn't directly translate to a reduction in body fat. Body fat reduction is a complex physiological process that involves a number of factors. Second, the human body needs a certain amount of high-quality fat in the diet every day. Eliminating fat from the diet is very risky to overall health and is very difficult to maintain for any length of time. This low-fat, low-protein and high-carbohydrate diet will create not only a state of low energy, but a feeling of constant hunger, hormonal imbalance and may even increase body fat as a result. The reasons for the consequences of this diet plan will become clear as you gain, throughout this book, a better understanding of nutrition.

Scenario 2

High-Protein, High-Fat, Low- or No-Carbohydrate Diet

This diet is almost the opposite of the high-carbohydrate diet described in Scenario 1. In this diet, carbohydrates are villainous. The idea is that by severely restricting carbohydrates, the body will burn protein and fat, thereby reducing body fat. Many find this diet easy to follow and easy to sustain because of the liberal fat and protein intake. The only foods that are limited are those high in carbohydrates. Dieters can eat as much as they want of any high-fat, high-protein food. On this diet people eat bacon, mayonnaise, prime rib, sausage, gravy—almost anything that doesn't seem like it belongs on a diet. What they don't eat are fruits, vegetables and whole grains. This diet also lacks an emphasis on eating quality fats and proteins. A typical menu for this dieter's day might look like this:

Breakfast	2 eggs 4 strips bacon coffee
Snack	2 slices cheese
Lunch	hamburger (no bun), with cheese lettuce salad with Ranch salad dressing
Snack	chicken salad with mayonnaise
Dinner	sirloin steak lettuce salad with Ranch salad dressing
Snack	cheddar cheese

If I severely restrict the carbohydrates in my diet (fruits, vegetables and whole grains), my body will burn fat and protein for energy, thus eating up all that unwanted body fat that I desperately want to be rid of. Limit carbohydrates, burn up more fat. Sounds great! But wait—you know the old saying, "If it seems too good to be true, it probably is." Like the high carbohydrate diet, this diet is also unbalanced. Doesn't common sense tell you that this eating plan cannot be healthy in the long run?

One reason for the popularity of high-protein, high-fat, low-carbohydrate diets is that the initial weight loss is very quick. Losing four to seven pounds in the first few days on this diet is very common; however, the initial weight loss is primarily due to a loss in water and muscle glycogen. When carbohydrates are restricted in your diet, the body looks to its carbohydrate reserves (glycogen) for fuel. Each gram of glycogen binds with four grams of water. The human body only holds approximately 500 grams of glycogen. Within just a few days of restricted carbohydrate intake, your carbohydrate reserves will be depleted, leading to a quick weight loss in the form of water. As you add carbohydrates back into your diet your glycogen will act as a sponge and absorb water, leading to a weight gain.

Another deterrent to this diet is the severe damage it can do to your health. If you restrict carbohydrate intake you will deny your body important vitamins, minerals, phytochemicals, fiber and food for the brain. The human brain needs approximately 400 calories per day (100 grams) from carbohydrates to function properly. Carbohydrate is the only source of fuel that the brain can use for energy. Once the body has used up its carbohydrate reserves (glycogen), it begins to look for other sources for energy. To fuel the brain, the body begins to break down fat and protein for energy. You may be thinking, "This is what I want. Use up my stored body fat as energy." Not so fast. Without carbohydrates, the body begins to convert fat into energy, but the by-product of this conversion is an abnormal biochemical called ketone bodies. The body tries to rid itself of these ketone bodies through increased urination and respiration (foul-smelling breath). With your fat cells going through this abnormal process to supply energy to the brain, future fat cells may be up to ten times more active in storing fat! To add even more fuel to the already unhealthy flame, your body also burns muscle protein for energy; as a result, you have less muscle. You don't want to lose muscle. The more muscle you have, the more calories your body burns at rest (your resting metabolic rate).

All things considered, this type of diet represents a serious risk to overall health and well-being. While it may deliver on the short-term promise of instant weight loss, it can't deliver long-term good health.

Scenario 3

Exchange/Low-Calorie Diet

This is a relatively balanced eating program where you have choices within similar groups of foods called "exchanges." It is a portion control diet plan that restricts calories by limiting the number and types of exchanges from each of the food groups. Dieters are sometimes encouraged to save their exchanges if they want to reward themselves with a certain type of disallowed food or want to splurge on a favorite food.

Lack of attention to the quality of foods is the main challenge of an exchange program. It is fairly well balanced among carbohydrates, proteins and fats, though it may err on the side of being somewhat low on quality fats. An exchange program gives little consideration to the nutritional composition or quality of foods the dieter consumes. There's a big difference between the quality of extra virgin olive oil and margarine, but both count as a fat exchange. The same is true in all food categories—some foods are higher quality and more nutritionally dense than others, even if they are approximately the same number of calories or count as the same number of exchanges. For example, a skinless chicken breast and a fat-free hot dog count as the same protein exchanges, but which do you suppose provides the highest quality protein?

These weight loss scenarios are just three of the myriad diet plans available, and all focus on reducing weight. Consider whether your only dieting goal is weight loss (decrease in percent of body fat). Might you also be seeking a way to maintain a high energy level? Do you want a diet that also helps you achieve optimal health? All three are worthy goals for a nutrition plan. Conventional diets directly address only weight loss, down-playing or ignoring optimal health and energy level concerns. With a new, Meal Patterning-inspired nutrition plan, all three goals are possible. You can reach your weight target, improve your energy and achieve optimal health.

Breakfast	cold cereal fruit skim milk toast w/fat-free margarine coffee
Snack	low-fat breakfast bar
Lunch	low-calorie frozen entree

Dinner	chicken breast
	steamed broccoli
	1/2 baked potato
	  with no-fat sour
	  cream

Snack	fat-free frozen yogurt

Chapter 3

Old vs. New Thinking

The only boundaries we have are in form.
There are no obstacles in thought.
— Dr. Wayne W. Dyer

Let's take a look at some pervasive old thinking about nutrition and compare it to newer, more contemporary ideas based on solid research.

Old Thinking

The Traditional Food Pyramid

Let's examine, visually, the differences between old ways of thinking about nutrition and the new thinking of Meal Patterning.

Food Guide Pyramid
A Guide to Daily Food Choices

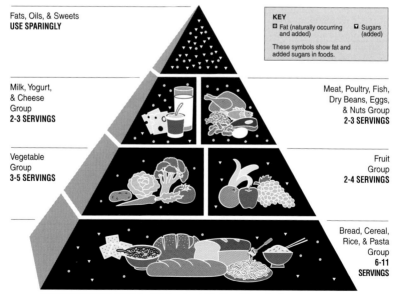

Fats, Oils, & Sweets
USE SPARINGLY

KEY
☐ Fat (naturally occurring and added)   ▼ Sugars (added)
These symbols show fat and added sugars in foods.

Milk, Yogurt, & Cheese Group
2-3 SERVINGS

Meat, Poultry, Fish, Dry Beans, Eggs, & Nuts Group
2-3 SERVINGS

Vegetable Group
3-5 SERVINGS

Fruit Group
2-4 SERVINGS

Bread, Cereal, Rice, & Pasta Group
6-11 SERVINGS

Source: U.S. Department of Agriculture/U.S. Department of Health and Human Services

The old thinking uses the traditional USDA food pyramid to guide daily food choices. The base of the food pyramid is reserved for carbohydrates—you are advised to eat six to eleven servings of bread, cereal, rice and pasta each day. The pyramid discourages fat and sugar consumption by placing them at the top of the pyramid.

A major fault of the pyramid is that it gives little consideration to the source or quality of foods. There is no distinction between good and bad fats, refined and unrefined carbohydrates and types of proteins. Pacific salmon, which is in the general protein category (meat, poultry, fish, beans, eggs and nuts) is a superior form of protein due to the healthy fat it contains. In the food pyramid, however, Pacific salmon is lumped together with hamburger, pork and even hot dogs. There is no recognition of the quality of the salmon over the many other types of proteins in the group.

The second problem with the USDA food pyramid is its lack of balance. Breads, cereal, rice and pasta form the base of the food pyramid with a recommended six to eleven servings each day. This is far too many carbohydrates for most people. The food pyramid also does not incorporate enough quality fats. Quality fats are essential for optimal health and should comprise 20-35 percent of your daily calories. The traditional food pyramid recommends limiting your fat intake.

> **66** When I started this adventure called "healthful living," I really didn't know what to expect from a fitness regime. Within weeks of beginning the Meal Patterning program, I began to feel a definite increase in my energy level and discovered the fun of both feeling and seeing muscles take shape and work with new strength and vigor.
>
> The recommended three meals and two balanced snacks kept me from feeling hungry or craving sweets. I was eating well—not dieting—and found that learning to make good food choices can easily become a lifestyle habit. A forty-pound weight loss and an improvement in my blood lipids was an added bonus. **99**
>
> **-Mary Kishler**

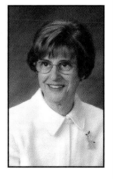

	1997	1998	2000
Cholesterol	278	237	210
LDL	169	133	107
HDL	80	91	93
Triglycerides	146	66	49
Cholesterol/HDL Ratio	3.5	2.6	2.3

New Thinking

The Food Target

I suggest replacing the old food pyramid with a food target to guide your daily food choices. The food target focuses on a balance of carbohydrates, proteins and fats while incorporating an assessment of the quality of these nutrients.

The new food target has the lowest nutrition foods on the outside of the target. These are the foods that contribute the least nutrition to the body and can be detrimental to your health. The most beneficial, most nutritious foods—those that make the body stronger—are closer to the center of the target. The idea behind the Meal Patterning program is to achieve balanced eating around the target and to concentrate your eating as close to the center of the target as possible. You will find foods in their most natural states closer to the center of the food target.

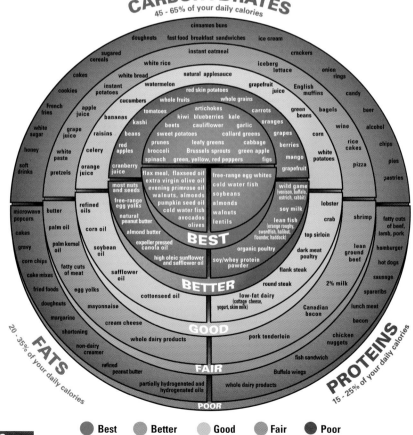

See full-size Food Target in back of book.

Old Thinking

Skip Meals to Lose Weight

A favorite trick of practiced dieters is to skip meals to lose weight. Many dieters starve themselves all day and eat only an evening meal. Let's look at the value of this technique by acquainting ourselves with Sumo wrestlers, who are experts at gaining weight. The Sumos have learned that it's not just what you eat that makes you gain weight, but also how, when, and what you do after eating. To gain weight, the Sumos are gorgers. They eat one or two meals of 3,500-4,500 calories each day. Immediately after eating, they take a two- to three-hour nap.

As an example, one budding Sumo wrestler initially weighed in at 350 pounds, and ate 6,000 calories a day spread over three meals. His typical calorie intake was 2,000 calories at breakfast, 2,500 at lunch and 1,500 calories at dinner.

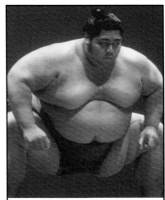

To gain more weight, he decided to change his approach to eating, or the patterns of his meals. After 18 months, he had gained almost 230 pounds while cutting his caloric intake by 2,000 calories a day. How did he do it? He simply adopted the life of established Sumo wrestlers. He decreased his frequency of eating, changing from three daily meals to one. He increased the quantity of food, eating 4,000 calories at his single meal, and he went to sleep immediately after eating.

How The Sumo Gained Weight
- Decreased his frequency of eating
- Increased the quantity of the meal
- Went to sleep immediately after eating

4,000 calories x 1 meal/day + Nap = 230 pound weight gain in 18 months

How is it possible to reduce the total calories consumed and the frequency of meals, and still gain weight? It is possible because of two processes the body uses to protect itself from starvation:

1. Your body protects itself from skipped meals. A key protector is lipoprotein lipase. Lipoprotein lipase is the key enzyme that stores fat to protect the body from starvation. When you decrease the frequency of meals or snacks, your lipoprotein lipase enzymes become more sensitive to storing calories. As the frequency of your meals decreases, your lipoprotein lipase enzymes begin to work overtime in an effort to store extra calories, in the form of fat, throughout your body.

2. After eating, the body's blood glucose level rises, initiating a release of the hormone insulin. Insulin opens cells to nutrients. Once the needs of the cells are met, the rest of the nutrients are stored as body fat. The increase in insulin levels leads to an increase in body fat stores as well as greater insulin resistance.

By the way, many Sumo wrestlers develop Type 2 diabetes by the age of 30 and many die in their late 40s.

New Thinking

Eat Small Meals Frequently

The adage of three square meals a day belongs in the old thinking category. New thinking balances your total calories evenly throughout the day in five or six small meals of roughly equal proportion.

Look closely at the difference in how these calories are consumed, and think back to the Sumo wrestlers and their gorging habits. Our old thinking would have us skip one or more meals, avoid snacking and then gorge at one meal, usually dinner. We're so hungry by then that we eat anything we can put our hands on quickly—candy, crackers, chips, cookies—and then eat dinner on top of these snacks.

New thinking evenly spaces meals throughout the day, including light snacks at mid-morning, mid-afternoon and evening. By increasing your frequency of eating, you will increase your metabolic rate, maintain a steadier blood glucose level, and reduce your chances of overeating at a given meal. Plus, you will not be hungry during the day. Other benefits to spacing out your meals are better focus all day (avoiding the typical 3:00 p.m. slump that

Meal	Old Thinking	New Thinking
breakfast	none	400 calories
snack	none	250 calories
lunch	500 calories	400 calories
snack	none	250 calories
dinner	1500 calories	550 calories
snack	none	150 calories
total	**2,000**	**2,000**

often leads to binge eating at dinner) and having a balanced sense of well-being and energy throughout the day and evening. Bottom line: You will just plain feel better and have a smaller waistline.

Old Thinking

Cut Calories to Lose Weight

Many people lose weight by reducing calories, only to gain the weight back and then some. Reducing the number of daily calories consumed is usually the first thing people do when they want to lose weight. Unfortunately, this is the wrong choice.

One of the fundamentals of long-term control of body fat is to maintain or increase lean muscle tissue. If you lose weight by restricting calories, a large percentage of your weight loss is often due to a loss of lean muscle tissue. As your lean muscle decreases, your body's ability to burn calories at rest (resting metabolic rate) decreases. Each pound of lean muscle tissue burns 60-70 percent more calories at rest than each pound of fat. So for every pound of fat that you replace with muscle, your body burns more calories (resting metabolic rate increases). That is why regular exercise is critical for long-term control of body fat.

A common weight loss approach is to determine the number of calories required to maintain your current weight and reduce the number of calories consumed accordingly. For example, if your body needs 2,000 calories per day to maintain your current weight, the theory is that by cutting back to 1,500 calories per day you should lose one pound per week (7 days x 500 calorie deficit per day = 3,500 calories = one pound of fat loss). Adding exercise to the plan is a bonus and calories burned through exercise should contribute to further weight loss. This approach seems pretty simple. Eat less, exercise more and watch the weight fall off. The truth is, it's not that simple.

The number of calories each person needs each day depends on many variables. The variables include activity level, frequency of meals, food quality, quantity of food at each meal, lean muscle tissue, food combinations, genetic factors and stress levels. It is possible to cut calories and still gain body fat. The amount of food, measured by number of calories you eat each day, is one factor in the weight loss equation, but it is not the best measurement for weight loss or good health.

With Meal Patterning, you will learn that calories are important, but the quality of food you eat, the combination of fat, protein and carbohydrate, and the frequency of eating have equal importance in the weight loss and good health formula.

New Thinking

All Calories Are Not Created Equal – Quality Counts

The old thinking that focuses on counting and restricting calories treats all calories as equal. A calorie-restriction program treats calories from bad fats and refined sugars the same as it does calories from high-quality protein, good fats and unrefined carbohydrates such as fruits and vegetables. Does this make sense to you?

Consider the following meals, both of which are approximately 500 calories	
• 1 piece chocolate cake	• 2 chicken breasts, • mixed green salad with flaxseed oil and balsamic vinegar, • 2 redskin potatoes with 1/2 tablespoon of extra virgin olive oil

Now consider the effect each meal has on your energy, mood, health and waistline during the three to four hours after you finish it.

Chocolate Cake	Chicken/Greens/Redskin Potatoes
• huge spike in blood glucose leading to a drop in energy	• small spike in blood glucose leading to sustained energy
• low energy, lethargic thought process, irritability, anxiety	• great energy, clear thought process, elevated mood
• spike in insulin, increased fat storage and more food cravings, adding to the waistline	• small release in insulin, less fat storage, reduced food cravings, leading to a lean, fit body
• poorly balanced, low in vitamins and minerals, high in poor fats and refined sugars, leading to poor health	• well balanced, high in vitamins, minerals, fiber, high-quality fats, leading to hormonal balance and optimal health

The quality of the foods you eat has an immense effect on your performance, health and well-being.

Imagine purchasing a $5 million race horse and then feeding it high-fat, low-quality foods. Worse, imagine feeding it these poor foods only once or twice a day, on schedule, regardless of whether it was hungry, had worked hard, or was expected to perform. Add inadequate rest, not enough water and limited or no exercise to the dietary neglect and you have a race horse with little or no chance of winning.

Old Thinking

Eliminate Fat from the Diet

Many old-fashioned diets reduce or eliminate fat entirely from the diet, based on the premise that all fats are bad. While it is true that fats are calorie-dense—a small amount of fat contributes a relatively large number of calories—it is not true that all fats are bad or should be avoided. There are four categories of fat: two categories to avoid and two categories to learn more about and incorporate sensibly into your diet.

- **Bad Fat #1:** Trans-fatty acids. These are the worst of the bad fats. Hydrogenating, or hardening, vegetable oils creates trans-fatty acids. Trans-fatty acids are very difficult for the body to break down and also impair the normal use of the good fats. Trans-fatty acids are found in foods like margarine, shortening, most crackers, packaged baked goods, fried foods, and microwave popcorn— to name just a few.

- **Bad Fat #2:** Saturated fats. Saturated fats are also classified as bad fats. Saturated fats increase your risk of coronary artery disease, diabetes and obesity. Major sources of saturated fats are fast foods, processed foods (which may also include trans-fatty acids), animal fats, whole dairy products, baked goods and tropical oils.

- **Good Fat #1:** Monounsaturated fats. These are neutral fats. The neutral, monounsaturated fats are good for cooking because they are stable at high temperatures, do not easily oxidize and taste great. Monounsaturated fats are found in olives, seeds, legumes, extra virgin olive oil, avocados, expeller pressed canola oil, high oleic safflower oil, natural peanut butter and almonds.

- **Good Fat #2:** Polyunsaturated fats. These are also known as Omega 3 and Omega 6 fats and are a source of essential fatty acids (EFAs). You should incorporate these good fats into your daily diet. Omega 3 and Omega 6 fats include marine oils from salmon, cod, tuna and trout, ground flaxseeds, flaxseed oil, walnuts, unrefined soybean oil, borage oil, evening primrose oil, pumpkin seed oil, legumes, raw nuts, seeds and leafy greens.

New Thinking

Cut Bad Fats and Incorporate Good Fats

Just like calories, not all fats are created equal. It is true that there is a predominance of fats in the typical American diet that are both dense with empty calories and contribute to poor health and disease. The bad fats are trans-fatty acids and saturated fats found in foods such as fatty meats, butter, margarine, and in many processed foods. These are the fats to avoid in your diet.

Good fats promote health and should be eaten daily. The benefits of good fats include:

- **Insulation of the body—providing thermoregulation**
- **Production of energy**
- **Protection of the body's major organs**
- **Maintenance of cell membrane structures**
- **Transportation of fat-soluble vitamins**
- **Hormonal balance**

Old Thinking

Eat Anything and Take Supplements

People interested in changing their health and eating habits have dramatically increased their use of dietary supplements. Unfortunately, much of this increase stems from the pursuit of a "magic pill" to take the place of a more sensible, and successful, approach. The marketing of such products is very convincing. Eat whatever you want with no exercise. Take this supplement and watch fat melt away. Take this supplement before bedtime and wake up thinner. These products produce, at best, only short-term results and, at worst, can be dangerous. Can you take that "magic pill" for the rest of your life? There is no such thing as a "magic pill."

New Thinking

Focus on High Quality Foods First

Supplements have their place and can be beneficial, even essential, for many people. But supplements are not the place to start your nutrition program. Meal Patterning begins with the heavyweights, the macronutrients: carbohydrates (CHO), proteins (PRO) and fats (FAT). These form the foundation of what we consume daily and have the largest impact on our overall health and well-being. Consuming **real** foods containing well-chosen carbohydrates, proteins and fats will have a much greater impact on our health than any supplement ever could.

Summary of Old and New Nutritional Thinking

My intent with this book is to help you focus on the five areas of new thinking and incorporate them into your daily life for improved health and performance. Here's a quick reminder of the differences between old and new thinking when it comes to nutrition.

Old Thinking	New Thinking
• Food pyramid	• Food target
• Skip meals to lose weight	• Eat small meals frequently
• Cut calories to lose weight	• Eat high-quality foods— all calories are not created equal
• Eliminate fat from the diet	• Eliminate bad fats and incorporate good fats
• Eat anything and take supplements	• Focus on eating quality food first

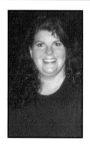 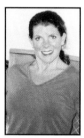

" Thanksgiving, 1999, I was looking through photo albums with my family after dinner. Flipping through the photo album, I realized there was a huge change in me, literally. My weight went from 160 lbs. to 258 lbs. in 3 years. I looked at those pages and could hardly believe it was me. I was disgusted, yet surprised. It was as if I was looking at pictures of someone else. From that moment my life would be forever changed.

I started by devoting time for myself at the gym six days a week. I read every nutrition/exercise book and magazine I could get my hands on. The book *Body for Life* suggested having your body fat percentage tested. I called Chris Johnson at the MAC. I was nervous to have someone else see my fat that closely; yet I knew and even said, "it won't be there for long." I started taking pictures of my progress every four weeks and I had my body fat tested then as well. Chris suggested two more books for me, *Meal Patterning* and *Eat Fat Lose Weight*, which I have read and followed to this day. Chris has been a great motivator and has given me information and knowledge that I am thankful for.

Two years later, 103 lbs. gone and 34 percent body fat gone, I now weigh 155. My body fat is at 22 percent. I cannot even describe the change in my energy level, I am much happier and feel great. I have not looked back once since I started this. I know this is not a quick fix. It is a continuing lifestyle change that I truly enjoy. "

-Lisa LaViolette

Macronutrients:
The Foundation of Meal Patterning

Every problem has in it the seeds of its own solution.
— Norman Vincent Peale

What are macronutrients? Macronutrients are carbohydrates, proteins and fats. Macronutrients are the fuel source for our bodies and minds.

- **Carbohydrates — Your Body's Energy Source**

- **Proteins — Your Body's Building Blocks**

- **Fats — Your Body's Healing Nutrients**

Consuming quality macronutrients in balance is the foundation of Meal Patterning. Throughout the next three chapters, I will help you understand how the macronutrients you consume affect your waistline, energy, mood, overall day-to-day performance and long-term health.

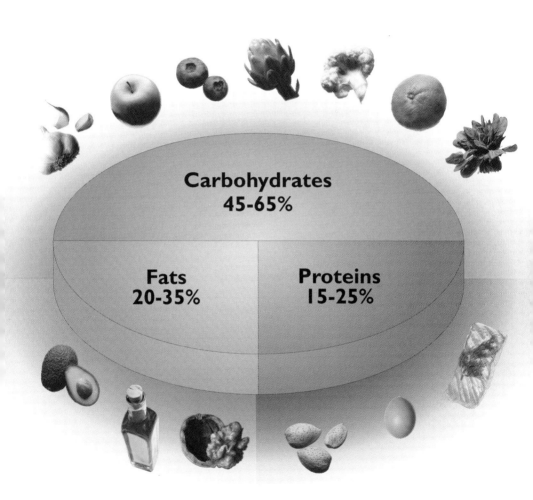

Carbohydrates
45-65%

Fats
20-35%

Proteins
15-25%

Chapter 4

Carbohydrates – Your Body's Energy Source

It's your attitude, not your aptitude, that determines your altitude in life.
– Unknown

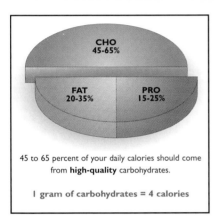

45 to 65 percent of your daily calories should come from **high-quality** carbohydrates.

1 gram of carbohydrates = 4 calories

What are carbohydrates? Carbohydrates are our energy foods. Carbohydrates are the primary source of food in our daily diet and provide us energy throughout the day. Carbohydrates are essential for optimal health and performance. They provide us with valuable vitamins, minerals, phytochemicals, fiber and energy for the brain and nervous system. The human brain needs 400 calories (100 grams) of carbohydrate per day to function properly. Carbohydrates are the only source of energy the brain can use, except during starvation.

Your goal each day is to consume between forty-five and sixty-five percent of your total calories from *quality* carbohydrates. Examples of carbohydrates include fruits, vegetables, breads, potatoes, cereals, pasta, legumes, juice, dairy products, soda pop and sugar. Some foods, such as cereals, bread and pasta contain a large amount of carbohydrates. Other foods, such as leafy greens, asparagus and broccoli contain a small amount of carbohydrates.

In our fast-paced, convenient, pre-packaged food society, carbohydrates fall on a continuum between refined and unrefined carbohydrates. Refined carbohydrates have been processed and stripped of essential nutrients. These refined carbohydrates are lacking in vitamins, minerals, phytochemicals and fiber. They include refined cereals, white bread, crackers, cookies, potato chips, candy, soda pop, honey and sugar, to name a few. Unrefined carbohydrates are foods in their most natural state. These include whole fruits, vegetables, whole grains and legumes. Consuming unrefined carbohydrates helps the body stay healthy and perform optimally.

Refined	The Carbohydrate Continuum	Unrefined
white bread	enriched wheat bread	100% whole grain bread
apple juice	natural applesauce	apple
catsup	salsa	tomato
sugared cereal	quick oats	100% rolled oats
corn syrup	creamed corn	whole kernel corn
orange drink	100% orange juice	orange

Fewer nutrients & fiber ← → More nutrients & fiber

Carbohydrate Chemistry

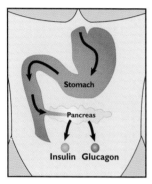

How Carbohydrates Work in the Body

Digestion breaks down the carbohydrates you consume into glucose. Digestion begins with the saliva in your mouth and continues through the stomach and intestines. As the carbohydrates are broken down, glucose passes into the bloodstream. The pancreas is the organ that controls blood glucose levels by unlocking two opposing hormones: insulin and glucagon.

When you eat, your blood glucose level begins to rise. In response to a rising blood glucose level, insulin is released to allow the cells to be fed. Insulin opens up the cells to admit blood glucose. The cells then use glucose for energy, or they store it as glycogen (carbohydrate) or fat. The cells call upon these stored nutrients when other nutrients are not available. When energy stores are full, excess blood glucose is stored as fat. Insulin is the key that opens up your cells for nourishment. Without insulin, your cells would starve to death.

Insulin is a fat-storing and hunger hormone. The ideal is to produce a sufficient amount of insulin and have your cells sensitive enough to open up easily. If you produce too much insulin in response to an increase in food intake (like the Sumo wrestlers), your body will store the excess carbohydrates, proteins and fats as body fat.

Insulin's antagonist is **glucagon**. Glucagon is the body's safety net in controlling blood glucose. It protects the body by preventing blood glucose from dropping too low. The pancreas releases glucagon as blood glucose drops. Glucagon directs the cells to release stored carbohydrate as glucose to raise your blood glucose level. Glucagon is a carbohydrate- and fat-releasing hormone.

Eating frequent small meals (150-400 calories per meal) throughout the day helps keep these hormones in balance. Remember, this is counter to the practice of many dieters who stimulate their pancreas to overproduce insulin by eating one or two large meals per day.

The Glycemic Index

It can be difficult to predict how certain carbohydrates affect blood glucose levels. Common sense would lead us to believe most refined, processed carbohydrates would cause a rapid rise in blood glucose and unrefined carbohydrates would have a smaller affect on blood glucose levels. In most cases this is all true, but the accuracy of determining how certain carbohydrates affect blood glucose can be greatly improved by using the Glycemic Index.

The Glycemic Index is a numeric tool that determines how individual carbohydrate foods affect blood glucose levels. Foods with a high Glycemic Index cause a large rise in blood glucose levels and foods with a low Glycemic Index have a smaller impact on blood glucose levels. Five factors determine how quickly carbohydrates in a food break down into glucose and enter the bloodstream.

1. **The structure of the carbohydrate:** There are three types of sugar structures: glucose, fructose and galactose. Glucose is found in grains, breads, pastas, cereals, vegetables and starches. Fructose is found in fruit. Galactose is found in dairy products. Glucose is the only sugar structure that is released directly into the bloodstream. Fructose and galactose are absorbed first by the liver, which converts them to glucose, slowing down their release into the bloodstream. The sugar in rice cakes, bagels and pasta enters the bloodstream very fast, while the sugar in apples, pears, ice cream and yogurt enters relatively slowly.

2. **How much the carbohydrate has been refined or processed:** Refined carbohydrates break down easily into glucose because they are stripped of valuable fiber. Then they quickly and easily enter the bloodstream. White bread has a high Glycemic Index compared to whole grain bread in which the fiber is still intact. Grape juice has a much higher Glycemic Index than whole grapes.

3. **The fiber content of the carbohydrate:** Fiber slows the release of carbohydrates into the bloodstream.

4. **The protein content of the food:** Protein slows the release of carbohydrates into the bloodstream.

5. **The fat content of the food:** Fat slows the release of carbohydrates into the bloodstream.

The Glycemic Index

The Glycemic Index is a tool measuring the rate at which a carbohydrate breaks down into glucose and enters the bloodstream. Foods high on the Glycemic Index break down more quickly than foods low on the Index. Foods broken down quickly cause a spike in blood glucose, a release in more insulin and eventually, a drop in your energy level.

Glycemic Index

Foods rated 70 and above are high glycemic foods

High					
glucose	100	pretzels	83	watermelon	76
corn flakes	92	rice cake	82	grape juice	75
mashed potatoes	92	sugared cereal	81	bagel	72
carrot	92	white bread	80	popcorn	72
white rice	85	jelly beans	78	millet	71
baked potato	85	doughnut	76	banana	70

Foods rated 56-69 are moderate glycemic foods

Moderate					
angel food cake	67	raisins	64	sweet corn	60
whole wheat bread	65	soft drink	63	white spaghetti	58
cantaloupe	65	bran muffin	60	peas	57

Foods rated 55 and below are low glycemic foods

Low					
orange juice	52	yam	37	avocado	0
brown rice	50	soy milk	36	leafy greens	0
grapes	50	chick peas	35	cucumber	0
grapefruit juice	48	split peas	32	raw broccoli	0
baked beans	48	lentils	29	walnuts	0
skim milk	46	yogurt	28	almonds	0
oatmeal (slow-cooking)	42	grapefruit	25	fish	0
orange	42	tomato	19	egg	0
rye bread	41	soybeans	18	chicken	0
apple	40	green or red pepper	0		

Notice that the majority of foods at the high end of the Glycemic Index are refined foods and most of the foods at the low end have little refinement and are in their most natural state. Try to choose foods in their most natural state. Avoid refined carbohydrates that, in addition to being high on the Glycemic Index, may be high in sugar, low in fiber, vitamins and minerals. Circumstances sometime warrant eating a food that may be high on the Glycemic Index. Under these circumstances, balancing that food with fats or proteins can slow the breakdown of the carbohydrate into glucose, thereby slowing its entrance into the bloodstream. Good examples are bananas and bagels. Using a banana in a smoothie, or eating a bagel with natural peanut butter slows the breakdown of these high glycemic carbohydrates.

The amount of carbohydrates also affects your blood glucose. Eating a half cup of carrots is going to have a much smaller impact on your blood glucose levels than eating a half cup of raisins. Carrots have a higher rating than raisins on the Glycemic Index (92 to 64), but the number of calories from a half cup of cooked carrots is 50 while the number of calories from a half cup of raisins is 230. It is important to understand the Glycemic Index in conjunction with the number of calories you consume. We will discuss more about quantity in Chapter 15.

Why Do We Crave Carbohydrates?

The Carbohydrate Black Hole

By eating too many or the wrong kinds of carbohydrates at one time, blood glucose may rise too rapidly, creating an insulin overshoot where the body releases more insulin than is needed.

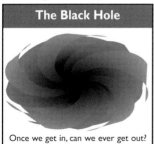

The Black Hole

Once we get in, can we ever get out?

Too much insulin causes blood glucose to plummet. When blood glucose levels drop, the brain feels deprived of food and signals for more energy. Because the level of insulin is too high, the brain is unable to stimulate glucagon, the hormone that releases carbohydrate from the liver and muscles. Remember, insulin and glucagon are opposing hormones, each fighting for the same space. If glucagon cannot release its reserves of carbohydrate, the brain signals you to eat more carbohydrates to offset the drop in blood glucose from the overabundance of insulin. Unfortunately, the ingestion of more refined carbohydrates further stimulates insulin production and the spiral continues into the **black hole**.

As a personal trainer I see this phenomenon in clients. They complain of low energy and the need for a quick picker-upper to increase their energy. When I look at their food logs, I see too many refined carbohydrates, little protein and virtually no fats. People experience highs and lows as their energy levels rise and fall due to their consumption of refined carbohydrates and the overproduction of insulin that results. The habit, or meal pattern, of most Americans for controlling their blood glucose is to pick themselves up with refined carbohydrates, or with caffeine in a soft drink or coffee.

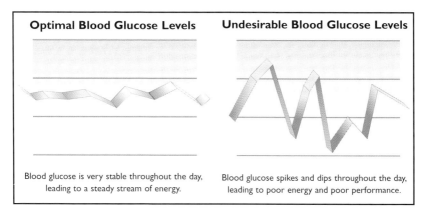

Optimal Blood Glucose Levels

Blood glucose is very stable throughout the day, leading to a steady stream of energy.

Undesirable Blood Glucose Levels

Blood glucose spikes and dips throughout the day, leading to poor energy and poor performance.

Insulin is a Hunger Hormone

Insulin is a powerful hormone that triggers humans to eat. Once insulin is over-produced by eating too many or the wrong types of carbohydrates, insulin becomes a very powerful hunger trigger.

Thanksgiving gives us a perfect example of how insulin works as a hunger trigger. The average American consumes 2,000 to 4,000 calories at a single meal on Thanksgiving . Within a short time, the nap syndrome kicks in: post-dinner drowsiness, just like the Sumo wrestlers who promptly go to sleep following their single big meal of the day. Upon waking, the first urge is to eat again. You probably are not craving that leftover broccoli. No, you most likely want a sandwich with lots of bread, mashed potatoes, stuffing or another piece of pie. This is the effect of the hunger hormone, insulin. As insulin levels rise to extreme heights after a very large meal, blood glucose will drop quickly, creating hunger for more refined carbohydrates.

Carbohydrates as Mood Regulators

When we become stressed or have low mood levels, we instinctively reach for comfort foods: refined, starchy carbohydrates. Eating carbohydrates, especially refined or starchy carbohydrates, increases the activity of serotonin.

Serotonin is a neurotransmitter used by the brain to communicate. Higher levels of serotonin regulate appetite and motivation and enhance mood. Serotonin has a calming affect on the brain. Consider that Prozac®, one of the nation's most prescribed anti-depressants, works by increasing serotonin activity.

By understanding the role carbohydrates play in your nutrition program, your health, energy, body fat and mood can all be under your control.

How Many Carbohydrates Should You Eat Each Day?

As you read further, I will show you how to moderate the effect of carbohydrates by adding a balance of proteins and fats to your diet.

Carbohydrates are essential for optimal health and well being. Choose carbohydrates in their most natural state (unrefined). Your goal should be to get 45-65 percent of your calories from unrefined carbohydrates. See guide on page 29 for carbohydrate intake compared to overall calorie intake.

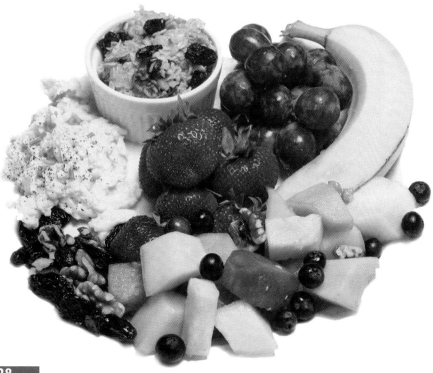

Recommended Carbohydrate Consumption Based on Daily Calorie Intake		
Total Calories	Grams of Carbohydrates	Number of Carbohydrate Calories
1,200	135-195	540-780
1,500	170-245	675-975
1,800	200-290	810-1170
2,000	225-325	900-1300
2,500	280-405	1125-1625
3,000	335-485	1350-1950

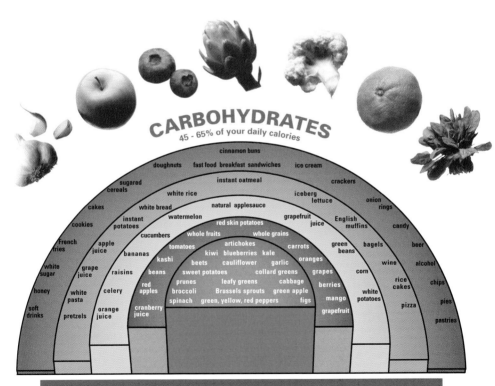

Reminder: Use the food target to guide your food choices.

Chapter 5

Proteins –
Your Body's Building Blocks

Work like you don't need money, love like you've never been hurt,
and dance like no one's watching.
— Ray Denning

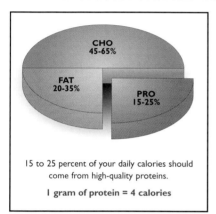

15 to 25 percent of your daily calories should
come from high-quality proteins.

1 gram of protein = 4 calories

While many of us are already eating enough protein, we all should consider the quantity, quality, and how frequently we eat protein throughout the day.

Protein is essential to life. It plays a role in every cell of the body. Proteins create hormones, maintain the immune system, build muscle, transport vitamins, and maintain our blood, skin and connective tissue.

Amino Acids

Our bodies break down protein into smaller nitrogen-containing units called amino acids. There are 22 amino acids: nine essential amino acids, and 13 non-essential amino acids. The body cannot manufacture essential amino acids, so we must get them through the foods we eat. If one or more of the essential amino acids is missing from our diet, a protein deficiency will develop.

Complete and Incomplete Proteins

Complete proteins contain all nine essential amino acids. Sources of complete proteins include eggs, meat, dairy products, poultry, fish and soy-based foods.

Incomplete proteins include some, but not all, of the essential amino acids. Foods that contain incomplete proteins include grains, rice, vegetables and beans. It is possible to combine different incomplete proteins to form complete proteins and thereby get all the essential amino acids we need.

When eaten together, the following combinations of foods make complete proteins that are easily absorbed by the body.

• corn and beans	• granola and yogurt
• rice and lentils	• oatmeal and milk
• pasta and bean salad or soup	• vegetarian chili (with beans)
• peanut butter sandwich	• bean soup and bread
• vegetable/tofu stir-fry	

What If You Don't Get All the Essential Amino Acids?

If your body is deficient in any one of the nine essential amino acids, it will begin to cannibalize the structural proteins of vital organs such as the liver and kidneys as well as its own muscle tissue to extract them. This is why a balanced diet is so critical in keeping the body strong and healthy.

Benefits of Protein

In addition to keeping the body strong and healthy, there are further benefits of eating enough protein.

• **Cell development:** Protein ensures your body receives appropriate amounts of the essential amino acids for cell development.

• **Increased energy:** Protein increases your energy level almost overnight. Protein helps to stabilize your blood glucose. You will not overproduce insulin when your blood glucose level is stable and you will enjoy greater energy consistency throughout the day.

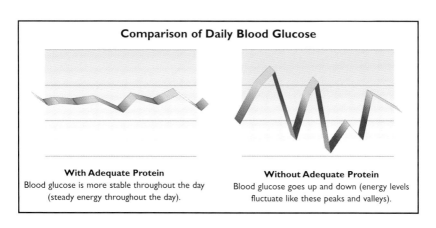

Comparison of Daily Blood Glucose

With Adequate Protein	**Without Adequate Protein**
Blood glucose is more stable throughout the day (steady energy throughout the day).	Blood glucose goes up and down (energy levels fluctuate like these peaks and valleys).

• **Reduced cravings for refined carbohydrates:** By adding protein to your daily diet, your cravings for carbohydrates, especially refined carbohydrates, will diminish.

• **Glucagon stimulation:** Glucagon is insulin's opposing hormone. Insulin is a fat/carbohydrate-storing hormone. Glucagon is a releasing hormone which aids in stabilizing blood glucose and boosting metabolism.

• **Improved brain power:** Adequate amounts of protein can improve cognitive skills, memory, focus and alertness. The first brain function to suffer the effects of age is memory. Memory begins to decline at about age 30 and loss of memory accelerates after age 40. To prevent this decline in memory and improve cognitive skills, focus and alertness, all nine essential amino acids must be consumed daily in adequate amounts.

What Kinds of Protein Should You Eat?

Try to incorporate only quality proteins into your nutritional program. Here's a list of good choices.

Soy-based Foods

Human beings have been eating soy for more than 5,000 years—so its health benefits are well established. Soy may be added to most foods and recipes, is neutral in flavor and is very high in plant-based protein. Soy is also rich in naturally-occurring isoflavones. Isoflavones are plant estrogens that may help fight cancer and reduce the risk of heart disease. The most powerful isoflavone, called genistein, appears to block key enzymes that tumor cells need to grow. Isoflavones also act as an estrogen modulator, aiding in balancing the hormone estrogen.

• **Soy milk:** Lactose-free soy milk is a great alternative to skim milk. It has a good ratio of carbohydrates (eight grams per serving), protein (seven grams per serving) and fat (four grams per serving). It tastes great on cereal or in your favorite smoothie drink. Look for calcium-fortified soy milk.

• **Tofu:** Perhaps the most well-known of the soy products, tofu is high in protein and looks a little like cheesecake. It is a healthy addition to almost any recipe (casserole, stir-fry, and in your smoothie drink).

• **Tempeh:** Tempeh is a fermented soybean patty made from whole soybeans that are soaked overnight. Tempeh is a great alternative to hamburger.

• **Soy-based meat substitutes:** Manufacturers of soy-based meat substitutes, such as soy chicken, soy meatballs and soy burgers, continually improve their products. You may be surprised at the variety and good flavor of these products. They are good to have on hand for quick and easy snacks or meals.

• **Soybeans:** Soybeans in the pod, known as edamame, can be steamed and eaten as a fresh vegetable. They are sweet, delicious and an excellent source of protein, fiber and isoflavones.

• **Soy nuts:** Soy nuts are an excellent source of protein, fat, fiber and isoflavones. They are sold in most natural food stores and come unsalted, salted and barbeque flavored.

• **Soy protein isolate:** Isolated soy protein is sold as a powder. It is very high in protein and is fat- and carbohydrate-free. You may use isolated soy protein in many ways. Add it to almost any recipe, cereal, pancakes, muffins or your favorite smoothie drink.

• **Texturized soy protein (TSP):** Texturized soy protein (TSP) is made from soy flour that is compressed. TSP is very high in protein, calcium, iron, isoflavones and zinc. TSP looks like granola and may be added to many recipes, such as meatloaf, chili, casseroles or hamburgers. Many cereals available at your local natural food store incorporate TSP.

How Much Soy Should You Eat?

According to the Food and Drug Administration, 25 grams of soy protein per day incorporated into a healthy diet can benefit most people. Although soy is a good source of protein and has many health benefits, consuming large amounts of soy is not recommended and could increase the risk of cancer, especially among breast and endometrial cancer survivors.

Eggs

When most people think of eggs, their first thought is that eggs are high in cholesterol and may cause heart disease. Yes, the egg yolk does contain 200 mg of cholesterol. For some people, a high cholesterol intake directly affects the amount of cholesterol in the bloodstream. But let's clear up a few misconceptions about eggs. The egg white itself is free of fat. Each egg white contains six grams of complete protein. The egg yolk is low in saturated fat and contains many other nutrients that are good for you, such as vitamins E and B, folic acid, choline (needed for proper brain functioning) and lecithin. Lecithin acts as a cholesterol-lowering agent and a natural emulsifier, helping prevent plaque build-up from blocking arteries. Eggs are also inexpensive and easy to prepare.

When buying eggs, choose only free-range or cage-free eggs. Free-range eggs are from chickens that are allowed to move about and graze freely on seeds, grains and insects. Consume egg yolks in moderation. Eggs can fit nicely into a diet for people who enjoy them.

Fish

Though generally a very good source of protein, not all fish are created equal. Orange roughy, halibut, swordfish, flounder and haddock are excellent sources of protein and very low in fat. Cold water fish such as salmon, trout, tuna, mackerel and bluefish are excellent sources of protein and high in heart-healthy Omega 3 fatty acids. When choosing cold water fish, such as canned tuna, select tuna packed in water and check the label for the brand with the highest content of healthy Omega 3 fats. You should be able to find brands with as many as five grams of this good fat. One or two servings of cold water fish per week will provide your body the wonderful benefits of Omega 3 fats. These benefits are discussed in greater detail in Chapter 6.

Poultry

• **Chicken:** White meat chicken is lower in saturated fat than dark meat chicken. Decrease the saturated fat content of chicken by removing the skin before cooking. As when choosing eggs, your best choice is organic, free-range chicken.

• **Turkey:** Turkey is much lower in saturated fat than most red meat. Like red meat, it is available in many forms—whole, or in parts, for roasting or baking, sliced for grilling, or ground as a delicious, healthy substitute for hamburger in soups, stews, pasta sauce, casseroles and your other favorite recipes.

• **Ostrich:** Ostrich is becoming a popular alternative to both red meat and other forms of poultry. It is low in saturated fat, high in protein, and is typically served as ostrich steaks or burgers. Ostrich is great for grilling and has excellent flavor.

Lean Red Meat

Most red meat contains high levels of saturated fat, which may lead to many health problems. However, the occasional serving of lean red meat can be part of a healthy, balanced diet and is a good source of iron. Red meat is also a complete protein. When choosing red meat, look only for lean cuts such as flank steak, top sirloin, round steak or beef tenderloin.

Most game meats are lean options when compared to traditional meat choices.

Buffalo and venison are examples of excellent meats popular with health-conscious consumers who want high-quality meat protein sources that taste good.

The Other White Meat?

Pork, along with red meat, may contain high levels of saturated fat. Choose lean cuts of pork such as pork tenderloin or lean pork chops.

Low-fat Dairy Products

Skim milk, low-fat cottage cheese, low-fat cheeses such as Feta, Mozzarella, and goat, along with non-fat yogurt are excellent sources of protein and calcium. Incorporate low-fat dairy products into your diet in moderation, allowing one or two servings per day.

Protein Supplements

If you are following a vegetarian diet or are just plain busy, protein supplements can be a beneficial, quick and easy addition to help balance your diet. The four types of protein supplements are whey, soy, egg albumin and milk protein isolates. Whey protein is the best selling protein supplement, followed by soy. Whey is made from dairy, and soy from soybeans. Both are excellent protein supplements. There has been some debate over which type of protein supplements is best, but any of the four available can provide an excellent source of supplemental protein to your daily nutritional program.

• **Whey.** Whey has been rated as having the highest biological value, which means it may yield more usable grams of amino acids than other protein supplements and it is very low in lactose. Whey is easy to mix and works well in a smoothie drink or added to cereal at breakfast. Whey is derived from milk. Look for 100 percent ion-exchanged whey protein isolate.

• **Soy.** Soy protein supplements are an excellent source of soy in your diet while also adding protein. Soy is a vegetable protein and is easy to mix. When choosing a soy protein supplement, look for "isolated soy protein." Look for Supro® isolated soy protein, non-GMO (Genetically Modified Soybean).

• **Egg Albumin.** Egg protein powder is not as popular as whey or soy, but is an excellent source of protein. Egg does not mix as easily as the other alternatives and does not have a pleasing taste.

• **Milk Protein Isolates.** Like whey, milk protein isolates have a high biological value, but contain lactose, which may upset the digestive systems of many people.

Choose only pure protein supplements, with no artificial sweetener and little or no added sugar (shown on the label as fructose or sucrose).

How to Use Protein Supplements

One complaint I get from many of my clients or seminar attendees is that it is challenging to eat frequently and that getting protein throughout the day may be difficult.

At breakfast, people may not have time to cook eggs, or the thought of having a piece of chicken is somewhat unappetizing. Or at work they just can't open up a can of tuna fish and gulp it down without smelling up the entire place! What can you do? Using protein supplements may be your answer to these challenges. In the morning, add a small amount of a protein powder to your favorite cereal. I add whey or soy to my oatmeal every day. It's quick and easy, and I like the taste. Just try it for a week and you will see. It stays with me for a few hours. I'm not hungry and have energy to spare.

During the day it can be difficult to find time to eat and especially to get a balance of protein. This is where a smoothie drink comes in. Instead of reaching for a prepackaged meal-replacement drink, make your own high-quality, healthy, balanced smoothie (include only the best quality protein, carbohydrates and fats). During the day, I make a smoothie drink with fruit, flaxseed oil, water and whey or soy protein. This allows me to eat frequently, keep my energy high throughout the day and get the balance of carbohydrates, proteins and fats I need to keep my body strong and healthy.

Protein/Energy Bars

There are many varieties of protein or energy bars available in the market today. It seems as though every day a new bar, with some new promise, is introduced. Protein/energy bars can be beneficial as a quick and easy snack when you are traveling or simply have a busy schedule and need some nourishment on the run. It's true that they are very convenient and manufacturers have greatly improved the taste of these bars. I caution clients against using these bars as meal replacements. They are a good, once-in-a-while, convenient substitute when other healthy options are impossible. They should *not* substitute for meals of real food. When choosing a protein or energy bar, be sure to read the label and pay close attention to three considerations.

- **Quality of the ingredients:** Avoid bars with fractionated or hydrogenated oils and those that are high in sugar.

- **Balance:** Choose a bar that is balanced with carbohydrates and proteins.

- **Taste:** Don't eat foods you don't like—it's unnecessary. There are many good-tasting bars on the market today. Find one that satisfies the other criteria and tastes good as well. Two of my favorites are the Odwalla™ and Cliff™ bars. Just remember that protein/energy bars should not be used consistently as meal replacements.

How Much Protein is Enough?

Eating adequate amounts of protein is not the same as overeating protein. Eating too much protein can be as damaging to the body as not eating enough. Getting more than 25 percent of your daily calories from protein may cause the body to become acidic. When amino acids (proteins) are broken down, they must be neutralized by buffering elements, namely calcium and magnesium. If your protein intake is too high, those buffering elements may become depleted which could lead to a decrease in bone mass. Eating too much protein also places stress on the liver and kidneys which have to work harder to rid the body of the by-products of excess protein metabolism.

Protein has tremendous nutritional benefits when balanced correctly in your diet. Your goal should be to get 15-25 percent of your daily calories from quality protein sources, spread evenly throughout the day.

Recommended Protein Consumption Based on Daily Calorie Intake		
Total Calories	Grams of Protein	Number of Protein Calories
1,200	45-75	180-300
1,500	56-94	225-375
1,800	68-113	270-450
2,000	75-125	300-500
2,500	94-156	375-625
3,000	113-188	450-750

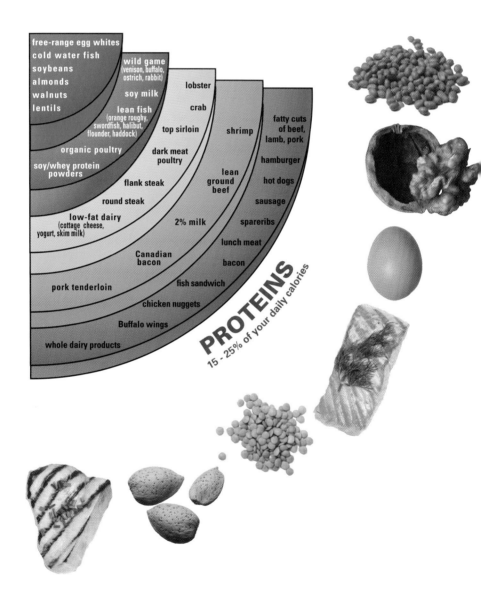

free-range egg whites
cold water fish
soybeans
almonds
walnuts
lentils

wild game
(venison, buffalo,
ostrich, rabbit)

soy milk

lean fish
(orange roughy,
swordfish, halibut,
flounder, haddock)

organic poultry

soy/whey protein
powders

low-fat dairy
(cottage cheese,
yogurt, skim milk)

pork tenderloin

whole dairy products

lobster

crab

top sirloin

dark meat
poultry

flank steak

round steak

2% milk

Canadian
bacon

fish sandwich

chicken nuggets

Buffalo wings

shrimp

lean
ground
beef

fatty cuts
of beef,
lamb, pork

hamburger

hot dogs

sausage

spareribs

lunch meat

bacon

PROTEINS
15 - 25% of your daily calories

Reminder: Use the food target to guide your food choices.

38

Chapter 6

Fats –
Your Body's Healing Nutrients

You pay the price, but you get what you pay for.

– Marie Fleming

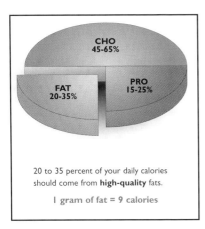

20 to 35 percent of your daily calories
should come from **high-quality** fats.

1 gram of fat = 9 calories

We are a nation obsessed with a fear of fat. 60 percent of Americans rank cutting fat as their number one nutritional concern. You cannot walk through the grocery store without seeing "fat and cholesterol free" plastered on every type of food imaginable. We have been led to believe that if a food has little or no fat, it must be okay to eat, and that foods containing fats should be avoided at all costs. This is flawed thinking. In this chapter you will learn to view fats in a whole new light.

In my Meal Patterning seminars, I spend a good deal of time explaining the benefits of eating quality fats and giving direction on how much to consume daily. Nonetheless, it never fails that immediately following the discussion of quality fats, a participant will approach me at the break to lament that extra virgin olive oil or natural peanut butter—which I just recommended—has 14 grams of fat per serving. My standard response is to ask if they had the same mind set when they looked at the box of oatmeal and saw 27 grams of carbohydrates per serving, or at the can of water packed tuna that has 20 grams of protein per serving. Until convinced about the importance of incorporating quality fats into the diet, people immediately look at the labels, see the amount of fat and wonder how I could possibly recommend that much fat be added to their diets.

I see the same mind set with personal training clients. A client may come to see me with the goal of lowering cholesterol, controlling diabetes or simply losing weight. I spend considerable time explaining the benefits of eating the right kinds of fats, show research, share testimonials and share my own experience with—and passion for—eating good fats. Clients with this information still often reject the idea of adding any type of fat to their diets.

We have been led to believe that all fats are unhealthy and will cause us to gain weight and become fat. True, fats do contain over twice the calories per gram (9 calories) as carbohydrates and proteins (4 calories). But consuming fat creates satiety, decreasing the desire to overeat. Consuming healthy fats can play a big role in controlling appetite and our overeating epidemic.

One conclusion that can be drawn from recent medical research is that you don't have to give up fat to lose weight or enjoy better health. In fact, the opposite is true. You should **not** give up all fat. Many calorie-restricted, weight-loss diets throw out the good fats with the bad fats, leaving dieters with a bland, low-energy, dissatisfying diet. Such a diet is virtually impossible to maintain over time and is unbalanced and unhealthy.

One of the primary goals of Meal Patterning is to help you distinguish between good and bad fats. It encourages eliminating the bad fats but promotes eating good fats so you will enjoy the performance and health benefits they provide.

Medical Research Supporting Good Fats

The definitive study showing the benefits of good fats is the Seven Countries Study, a 15 year study involving 12,000 men from Greece, Italy, Netherlands, Finland, Japan, Yugoslavia and the United States. This study concluded that the people of the Greek island Crete (eating a diet virtually unchanged since 4,000 B.C.) had the lowest death rates from cancer and heart disease. Crete had half the death rate from cancer and one-twentieth the death rate from heart disease of the United States. What is unique about the Cretan diet?

First, the overall fat intake is high—35 percent of calories come from fat. Second, the types of fat consumed are much different than the types of fat consumed in the United States. The Cretan diet is low in trans-fatty acids and saturated fats (bad fats) and high in monounsaturated fats and Omega 3 fatty acids (good fats).

How Does the U.S. Compare?

In the United States we continue to increase our intake of trans-fatty acids and saturated fats from processed snacks and animal products. Americans are consuming too many refined Omega 6 fats and not enough Omega 3 fats.

As a result of our poor eating habits, we have seen a dramatic rise in

- obesity
- auto-immune diseases
- arthritis
- diabetes (type 2)

- heart disease
- cancer
- depression
- dementia

Where Have We Gone Wrong?

Since the early 1960s we have slowly decreased our percentage of calories coming from fat, especially good fats. The more refining that goes into producing food, the more quality (good fat) is stripped away. We are a nation of convenience eaters. In return, we get unhealthy, refined, convenient food sources. Our entire food supply has been affected by our demand for convenience and packaged foods. In his book *Fast Food Nation*, Eric Schlosser explains, "Americans spend more on fast food than they spend on higher education, personal computers, computer software, new cars, movies, books, magazines, newspapers, videos, and recorded music combined." McDonald's® is the nation's largest purchaser of beef and potatoes and the second largest purchaser of chicken.

Why do food manufacturers and the fast food industry use poor quality fat in packaging and preparing food? **Money. First,** refined soybean or corn oil are very inexpensive oils that are used in thousands of food products to enhance taste. **Second** is increased shelf life of food products. Poor-quality fats extend the shelf life of a food product. **Third,** and most important, good fats are more expensive and have shorter shelf lives so manufacturers are driven by cost considerations to use low-quality, cheap fat in processing foods. Let's look at a few examples.

Butter vs. Margarine

Margarine is nothing more than hydrogenated oil—one of the poorest quality fats you can eat. Hydrogenation is the most common method for changing a polyunsaturated fat into a trans-fatty acid. Manufacturers start with a cheap oil (such as corn or soybean oil) and process it through hydrogenation (high heat with a metal catalyst) which changes the oil into a hardened fat or trans-fatty acid. Hydrogenation allows manufacturers to use cheap, low-quality oils and process them into a product designed to compete with butter. The low cost of raw materials allows the margarine to be sold at a much lower price than butter. Manufacturers spend large sums of money on advertising campaigns to convince Americans that margarine is healthier than butter, which simply isn't true.

Soft Cookies

At one time I worked as a route salesperson for a snack food company. I handled a variety of snack foods, including potato chips, pretzels and packaged soft cookies. Potato chips and pretzels have a four to six week shelf life before being returned as stale. Packaged soft cookies, on the other hand, have a shelf life of over 36 months—**three years!** How can the shelf life of soft cookies be so long? The cookies are loaded with trans-fatty acids. If trans-fatty acids can preserve a bag of cookies for three years, think about the effect they have on your body once they are consumed.

These are just two examples of how bad fats make their way into our cupboards and onto our dinner tables. In our society, we have to search for good fats while working overtime to avoid bad fats.

Why Is Eating Good Fats So Essential to Optimal Performance and Good Health?

The human body is made up of billions of cells. Each cell has a specific job to do and is in a constant state of change. On the most basic level, fat helps form the membrane that surrounds each of your cells. This membrane controls which elements enter and exit the cell. This is one of the major functions of the body that is threatened by eating trans-fatty acids (bad fats). Trans-fatty acids interfere with normal fat metabolism by crowding or pushing out essential fatty acids (Omega 3) from cell membranes. This makes the cell less fluid, less permeable, and reduces the number and sensitivity of the insulin receptors.

A compromised cell membrane is a major factor in Type 2 diabetes. When insulin approaches a cell and tries to open it up to allow nutrients to enter, it has a tougher time doing its job if trans-fatty acids have made the outer membrane of the cell less permeable to insulin and reduced the sensitivity and number of insulin receptors. The cell becomes insulin resistant.

Eating good fat promotes cell permeability and helps to satisfy your hunger. Fat content in food causes the release of a hormone called cholecystokinin (CCK) from the stomach. CCK alerts the brain that you are satisfied. Without sufficient fat, you are more likely to overeat. Fats also slow down the digestion of carbohydrates and proteins so that there is a more sustained release of nutrients into the blood, resulting in a stable energy level.

According to *Fats that Heal, Fats that Kill* by Udo Erasmus, the health benefits of eating good fats include:

Decreases	Improves
inflammation	the immune system
arthritis symptoms	brain development, cognitive skills, focus
cancer incidence	skin, hair and nails
migraine headaches	absorption of vitamins
post-menopausal symptoms	weight loss
depression	"brown fat" for body temperature regulation
constipation	cardiovascular health
high blood pressure	hormonal balance
cholesterol	overall health and well-being
platelet aggregation	ADHD (attention deficit hyperactivity disorder)

CAUTION: Consuming too much fat, including good fats, may lead to weight gain and hormonal imbalance.

> 66 Exercise and diet had long been a part of my lifestyle to keep fit and pass the frequent physicals required to keep my commercial pilot license. I thought I had a pretty good handle on living healthy. Last year, when the doctor checked my blood pressure on a routine visit he was alarmed at the numbers and wanted to put me on medication immediately to bring it down. I wanted to try something else first. I had attended one of Chris Johnson's Meal Patterning seminars the year prior and I felt there might be a nutritional solution for improving my blood pressure.

> After a few months of strict adherence to the program, my blood pressure was lower than at any time in my life. My cholesterol was down by over 40 points. I have maintained CJ's recommended plan and my health, energy and ability to sleep have improved. Associates from as far away as Fairbanks, Alaska, have heard how this has improved my life. I have purchased over 20 of Chris's books so that these people can follow the program with similar results. It feels wonderful to be this fit at my age and to be able to pass this along to my friends. Our fast-paced, pre-packaged lifestyle is not what the "doctor ordered" to keep us fit. Meal Patterning identifies the essentials of making the body run efficiently. I'm glad it's part of my life. 99   **- John DeCarli**

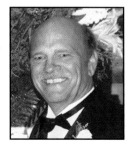

The Categories of Fats

Trans-fatty Acids

These are the worst of the bad fats. Hydrogenating, or hardening, vegetable oils creates trans-fatty acids. As noted earlier, the food industry widely uses transfats because they are inexpensive, improve taste and increase shelf life.

Trans-fatty acids are difficult for the body to break down and may impair the normal use of good fats by hardening the cell membrane. Trans-fatty acids raise LDL (bad) cholesterol and lower HDL (good) cholesterol, pushing both the bad and good blood fats in the wrong direction. Today, average Americans consume 20 percent of their calories from trans-fatty acids. Studies show that there is **no acceptable level** of transfat.

Unless we are vigilant, it is easy to consume trans-fatty acids because they are hidden in almost all processed foods. Trans-fatty acids are found in margarine, shortening, doughnuts, French fries, pound cake, most crackers, most potato chips and chip-like snacks, packaged soft cookies, most other packaged cookies, most packaged baked goods of any kind, and microwave popcorn. Look at the labels on the food you buy. Any time "**partially hydrogenated**" appears on a food label, the product contains trans-fatty acids.

Trans-fatty acids are such a serious health risk, the Food and Drug Administration will soon require that all food labels list them.

Saturated Fats

Though not quite as detrimental to your health as trans-fatty acids, saturated fats are still bad fats and should be avoided. A saturated fat is one that contains a significant amount of saturated fatty acids. Most saturated fats are solid at room temperature except for tropical oils such as coconut, palm and palm kernel oils.

The body recognizes saturated fats and can process these fats easily, compared to trans-fatty acids. The negative impact of saturated fats is similar to that of trans-fatty acids; they increase your risk for obesity, heart disease and diabetes. Saturated fats raise your bad cholesterol (LDL), but do nothing to affect your good cholesterol (HDL).

Animal products such as meat, eggs and dairy, as well as most seeds and nuts, all contain some saturated fats. The amount of saturated fat in food depends a great deal on what animals were eating and how they were raised.

For example, wild game such as buffalo has a much lower saturated fat content than most beef. Eggs from free-range chickens have less saturated fat than eggs from chickens that are raised in cages. An important principle in evaluating your food choices in all categories is to choose foods that are as natural as possible. When considering saturated fats in animal products, evaluate how the source of fat, the animal, was raised. The best quality saturated fats will come from those animals raised under the most natural conditions. To decrease the amount of saturated fat in the diet choose only the leanest cuts of beef, pork, poultry, wild game and low-fat dairy products.

Almost all nuts and seeds have some saturated fat content—some a little less, some a little more. Most nuts and seeds are an excellent source of fat, protein, and fiber. It is important to control serving sizes, however, in order to limit the amount of saturated fat, total fat and excess calories. Eat raw, not roasted, nuts.

Fractionated Fats

An emerging category of fat within the saturated fats is fractionated oils. Many of the protein bars with chocolate coatings use fractionated oils. Fractionation gives oils the same properties as hard oils (tropical, animal or hydrogenated oil), which make chocolate smooth and creamy. The label reads differently, but the negative effects to your health are similar to those of using tropical or hydrogenated oils.

Monounsaturated Fats (Omega 9 Fats)

Monounsaturated fats (also known as Omega 9 fats) play an important part in your balanced diet. Monounsaturated fats contain the fatty acid known as oleic acid.

Health Benefits of Monounsaturated Fats

Monounsaturated fats protect the arteries from cholesterol buildup, reduce the risk of breast cancer, accentuate the effect of Omega 3 fatty acids in the blood and help in the formation and development of all cell membranes, which is important for cell, tissue and organ health. One of the reasons monounsaturated fats are so protective against heart disease is that they lower LDL (bad cholesterol) while they maintain or even raise HDL (good cholesterol) levels—the best of both worlds. No other fat has this effect.

Monounsaturated fats are preferred over polyunsaturated fats for cooking because they have a single double-bond between their carbon atoms, making them stable at high temperatures, not easily oxidized and great tasting. Any time a recipe calls for oil, use only monounsaturated oils.

Where Do You Find Monounsaturated Fats?

Monounsaturated fats are found in olives, extra virgin olive oil, expeller pressed canola oil, avocados, avocado oil, almonds, almond butter, almond oil, peanuts, natural peanut butter, pistachios, pecans, cashews, hazelnuts and macadamia nuts. Monounsaturated fats are also found in high oleic expeller pressed safflower and sunflower oils. When choosing snacks like chips or crackers, look for those prepared with high oleic expeller pressed safflower or sunflower oils.

What to Look For When Buying Oils Made From Monounsaturated Fats

The process of refining affects oils and other products made from monounsaturated fats. Refining is increasingly prevalent in many foods. Producers of oil products use refining techniques to improve profits without regard to the negative effect they have on the products (and us!). Olive oil is a refined oil. Virgin olive oil is a better choice because it is less refined. Extra virgin olive oil is even better. To be called extra virgin means the oil is from the first pressing, is the highest quality, and has been extracted under strict adherence to specific guidelines. If olives are damaged or bruised, they begin to spoil and the oil pressed from them is of such poor quality that it must be refined, degummed, bleached and deodorized, resulting in olive oil that is equivalent in quality to cheap, mass-produced, mass-marketed oils. The processes used in mass-produced oils remove and strip many of the essential nutrients that provide critical health benefits. So, choose only extra virgin olive oil and other high-quality, unrefined oils. Store all your monounsaturated fats at room temperature in dark containers or in the cupboard .

How Much Monounsaturated Fat Should You Eat?

Approximately 15 percent of your daily calories should come from monounsaturated fats, roughly half of your total fat intake. If you consume 2,000 calories per day, approximately 300 calories, or 30 grams, should come from monounsaturated fats. 30 grams of monounsaturated fat is equivalent to three tablespoons.

For example, 300 calories of monounsaturated fats could be consumed by
• adding 1 tablespoon of natural peanut butter or almond butter to a piece of whole grain toast.
• using 1 tablespoon of extra virgin olive oil and 1 tablespoon balsamic vinegar as your salad dressing.
• adding 1 tablespoon extra virgin olive oil to your small bowl of air-popped popcorn.

Polyunsaturated Fatty Acids–Essential Fatty Acids

Polyunsaturated fats include essential fatty acids. This means we must obtain them from the foods we eat and they are necessary for the proper function of our bodies.

At a microscopic level, polyunsaturated fatty acids have two or more double-bonds in their carbon chains. The more double-bonds on the carbon chain, the more unsaturated the oil. Flaxseed oil and fish oil are the most unsaturated of all oils. All polyunsaturated oils are liquid at room temperature and remain liquid when refrigerated. We will discuss these oils in greater detail later in this section.

In the past, we believed that any type of polyunsaturated fat was healthy, with little distinction between types of polyunsaturated fatty acids. We now understand that polyunsaturated fats fall into two distinct groups: Omega 3 and Omega 6 essential fatty acids, each aiding specific functions in the body. The type of refinement or processing is very important with regard to the benefits of these fats.

Omega 3 Essential Fatty Acids

Omega 3 fats are the superstars of the good fats and make the body strong and healthy. The primary fatty acid in the Omega 3 family is alpha-linolenic acid (LNA). LNA is found in green leafy vegetables, flaxseeds, flaxseed oil, walnuts, brazil nuts, expeller pressed canola oil and pumpkin seeds. Flaxseeds and flaxseed oil are the *richest* sources of LNA.

Omega 3 Family

Alpha-Linolenic Acid (LNA)
(found in ground flaxseeds, flaxseed oil, walnuts, walnut oil, brazil nuts and leafy green vegetables)

your body converts LNA into:

Eicosapentaenoic Acid (EPA)
(EPA is also found in fish oil)

your body converts EPA into:

Docosahexaenoic Acid (DHA)
(also found in fish oil)

There are three levels of Omega 3 breakdowns, or conversions, in the body. LNA converts to one of two other types of fatty acids, depending upon its breakdown pathway. LNA is converted into eicosapentaenoic acid (EPA) and then into docosahexaenoic acid (DHA). Scientists became aware of the wonderful health benefits of EPA and DHA when Danish physicians observed that Greenland Eskimos had exceptionally low incidences of heart disease and arthritis, despite the fact that they consumed a high-fat diet. The type of fat the Greenland Eskimos were consuming was high in EPA and DHA, found in cold water fish such as salmon, trout, tuna, mackerel, herring and in fish oils.

People attending my Meal Patterning seminars often ask, "If I eat Omega 3 fats, such as flaxseed oil, which is high in LNA, do I also need to consume cold water fish or fish oil supplements which are high in EPA and DHA?"
For most healthy adults, LNA can be converted into EPA and DHA efficiently; however, the conversion is quite inefficient in many elderly, some infants and children, and those with metabolic diseases such as diabetes. These individuals must consume cold water fish once or twice a week to get adequate amounts of EPA and DHA.

Benefits of Consuming Omega 3 Foods

Hormonal Balance With Omega 3 Fats

Polyunsaturated fatty acids are important for creating hormonal balance in the body. Both the Omega 3 and Omega 6 fats work in the body by forming short-lived, hormone-like substances called prostaglandins. Prostaglandins regulate metabolic processes throughout the body at the cellular level. They control cellular communication and are essential in regulating the immune, reproductive, central nervous and cardiovascular systems.

Healthy Heart With Omega 3 Fats

Prostaglandins formed from Omega 3 fats aid the cardiovascular system by reducing constriction of blood vessels and decreasing the stickiness of the blood, making it less likely to clot. Eating too much bad fat (trans-fatty acids and saturated fats), and/or the wrong balance of polyunsaturated fats (too much Omega 6 and not enough Omega 3), will likely create a prostaglandin imbalance.

Omega 3 fats protect the heart by helping to prevent atherosclerosis, angina, heart attack, congestive heart failure, arrhythmias, stroke and peripheral vascular disease. Omega 3 fats help to maintain elasticity of artery walls, prevent blood clotting, reduce blood pressure and stabilize heart rhythm.

Your Brain Needs DHA

The Omega 3 fat docosahexaenoic (DHA) is the building block of human brain tissue and is abundant in the grey matter of the brain and the retina of the eye. Low levels of DHA have recently been associated with depression, memory loss, dementia and visual problems. DHA is particularly important for fetal and infant development. The DHA content of an infant's brain triples during the first three months of life. Optimal levels of DHA are, therefore, crucial for pregnant and lactating mothers. Unfortunately, the average DHA content in breast milk in the U.S. is the lowest in the world, most likely due to our failure to consume enough Omega 3 fats. Dr. Barbara Levine, Professor of Nutrition in Medicine at Cornell University, sounds the alarm concerning the inadequate intake of DHA by most Americans. Dr. Levine believes that common health problems in the U.S., such as postpartum depression, attention deficit hyperactivity disorder (ADHD) and low IQs, are linked to low DHA intake. Dr. Levine also points out that low DHA levels have been linked to low brain serotonin levels. Serotonin is the "feel good" neurotransmitter that is boosted by antidepressants such as Zoloft® and Prozac®.

Weight Loss With Omega 3 Fats

Omega 3 fats help weight loss in three important ways
1. Omega 3 fats increase metabolic rate, oxidation rate and energy production. Your body becomes more metabolically active and the rate of calorie expenditure increases.
2. Omega 3 fats improve your energy level, which makes you feel like being more active. You feel good and want to move your body more.
3. Omega 3 fats keep you satisfied, create a feeling of fullness and help control appetite and food cravings.

Where Do You Find Omega 3 Fatty Acids?

When I look at a typical client's food log, I rarely see adequate consumption of Omega 3 fatty acids. This is common among Americans who are eating more and more refined foods. It is a challenge to get enough Omega 3 fatty acids unless you know where to look. I tell clients, "You must search for Omega 3 fats." Why is that? Because foods that contain Omega 3 fatty acids spoil quickly. The more unsaturated a fat, the more fragile it is. Omega 3 fatty acids deteriorate with exposure to heat, light and oxygen. It stands to reason, then, that foods on grocery shelves with long shelf lives will not contain Omega 3 fats. There are, however, excellent sources of Omega 3 fatty acids available.

Flaxseeds. Flaxseeds are tiny, hard seeds, either gold or brown, that are loaded with Omega 3 fatty acids. The seeds themselves are not digestible, so to reap the wonderful health benefits of the Omega 3 fatty acids, the seeds must be ground into flaxmeal or pressed into flaxseed oil. Flaxseeds are inexpensive and are an excellent dietary fiber source. Flaxseeds contain lignans, which have anti-viral, anti-fungal, anti-bacterial and anti-cancer properties. Lignans are found in the seed coat. Only two percent of the lignans end up in the oil. "Lignan Rich" flaxseed oil is simply flax oil with fine seed material that typically settled to the bottom. If you want the benefits of lignans, use fresh ground seeds. Flaxseeds may be used on salads, cereals or in baking. Whole flaxseeds are high in fiber and help curb appetite.

Flaxmeal. Flaxmeal is ground flaxseeds. Flaxmeal is sold in health food stores, but I recommend that you purchase flaxseeds and grind your own meal in a coffee grinder to ensure that you are consuming fresh flaxmeal. Flaxseeds have a two year shelf life but flaxmeal can only be stored for two to three months. Once you've ground the flaxseeds, store the meal in a dark, airtight container in the refrigerator. Flaxmeal may also be frozen. Flaxmeal may be added to a variety of foods such as cereal, salads, smoothies and yogurt, and adds a nutty flavor. The recommended daily serving of flaxmeal is 2-1/2 tablespoons per day per 100 pounds of body weight.

Flaxseed Oil. An overwhelming amount of research has been done on the benefits of flaxmeal and flaxseed oil. Ground flaxmeal and flaxseed oil are the richest sources of Omega 3 fatty acids (LNA). You will find flaxseed oil in the refrigerated section of your local health or natural foods store. Flaxseed oil must be refrigerated and you should pay close attention to the date on the container—it has a shelf life of only two to three months. Do not heat or cook with flaxseed oil as heat destroys the Omega 3 fats. Flaxseed oil may be added to cereal, smoothies, yogurt, cottage cheese or drizzled on salad—be creative with it. When traveling, you may substitute flaxseed oil capsules for flaxseed oil, but it will be more expensive and may require a dose of up to 12 capsules, depending on your size. The recommended daily serving of flaxseed oil is one tablespoon, or six flaxseed oil capsules, per 100 pounds of body weight.

Form	Health Benefit	Use	Storage
Flaxseeds	Great source of dietary fiber and helps to curb appetite.	Sprinkle 1 to 2 Tbs. on cereal, salads or yogurt or use for baking.	Store at room temperature for up to 1 year.
Flaxmeal	Provides the most breast cancer-fighting lignans of any food. (If they're not ground, the seeds can't provide the lignans.)	Sprinkle 1 to 2 Tbs. on cereal, salads, in smoothies or add to your favorite muffin recipe.	Store in airtight container in refrigerator. May also be frozen.
Flaxseed Oil	Best source of alpha-linolenic acid, which fights heart disease, breast cancer and depression.	Add to cereals or salads, drizzle over bread or add to favorite smoothies, but don't use for cooking (heat breaks it down).	Buy refrigerated oil, and store in the refrigerator for 4 to 6 weeks. Discard if it smells "fishy" or "painty".

> "Wherever flaxseeds become a regular food item among the people,
> there will be better health."
> — Mahatma Gandhi

There are many other sources of Omega 3 fatty acids (LNA) such as walnuts, butternuts, brazil nuts, filberts, walnut oil, pumpkin seeds, pumpkin seed oil, hemp oil and soybeans. Many of these nuts and oils contain Omega 3, Omega 6 and monounsaturated fats. Leafy green vegetables also contain small amounts of LNA.

Wonderful Fish Oils

As stated earlier, eicosapentaenoic (EPA) and docosahexaenoic (DHA) can be manufactured by healthy cells from alpha-linolenic acid (LNA), which is found in great quantities in flaxseed meal and flaxseed oil. Your body, however, may not be very efficient in this process and degenerative conditions can impair the body's ability to make EPA and DHA from LNA. To directly get EPA and DHA into your body, take advantage of the wonderful benefits of fish oil.

The richest sources of EPA and DHA are cold water fish such as salmon, trout, mackerel, sardines, tuna and bluefish. To maintain the health benefits of EPA and DHA, you should eat cold water fish at least once a week.

Fatty Fish	Lean Fish
Salmon	**Flounder**
🐟🐟🐟🐟🐟 🐟🐟🐟🐟 (9)	🐟🐟 (2)
Mackerel	**Haddock**
🐟🐟🐟🐟 🐟🐟🐟 (7)	🐟 (1)
Trout	**Swordfish**
🐟🐟🐟🐟🐟 (5)	🐟 (1)
Tuna	**Orange Roughy**
🐟🐟🐟🐟 (4)	🐟 (Less than .01 g)
	🐟 = 0.2 g of heart saving Omega 3's

Unlike chicken and turkey, high-fat, cold water fish should be prepared with the skin on. Salmon and mackerel provide the greatest amount of Omega 3s. If you are opposed to eating these fish regularly, you may supplement your diet with fish oil capsules.

How Much Omega 3 Fat Should You Eat?

Make an effort to get one or two servings of unrefined, quality Omega 3s each day. Use 2-1/2 tablespoons of flaxmeal or one tablespoon of flaxseed oil per 100 pounds of body weight daily, and one or two servings of cold water fish per week.

Omega 6 Essential Fatty Acids

The second type of polyunsaturated fat is comprised of Omega 6 fatty acids. The primary fatty acid in the Omega 6 family is **linoleic acid (LA)**. Vegetable oils such as corn, cottonseed, safflower, sunflower, soybean, pumpkin seed and sesame seed all contain linoleic acid. It is also found in many nuts, seeds and leafy greens. Animal sources of Omega 6 fatty acids include lean meats, organ meats and mother's milk.

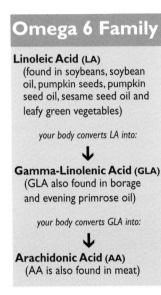

Omega 6 Family

Linoleic Acid (LA)
(found in soybeans, soybean oil, pumpkin seeds, pumpkin seed oil, sesame seed oil and leafy green vegetables)

your body converts LA into:

↓

Gamma-Linolenic Acid (GLA)
(GLA also found in borage and evening primrose oil)

your body converts GLA into:

↓

Arachidonic Acid (AA)
(AA is also found in meat)

Like the Omega 3 fatty acid family, which converts LNA to EPA and DHA, the primary Omega 6 fatty acid converts into two fatty acids, gamma-linolenic acid (GLA) and arachidonic acid (AA).

Like the Omega 3 family, the Omega 6 family contains essential fatty acids. The body cannot produce these essential fatty acids, so they must come from the food we eat.

Health Benefits of Omega 6 Essential Fatty Acids

As with Omega 3 fats, Omega 6 fats are essential for optimal health. Omega 6 fats are necessary for production of prostaglandins, the short-lived, hormone-like substances that regulate most of the body's life-sustaining systems. The body produces prostaglandins from the essential fatty acids we consume each day.

The Body's Good Fat—Brown Fat

Our bodies have two types of fat cells, white fat and brown fat. White fat is the fat under your skin that insulates the body and is used for energy. This is the fat most of us are trying to lose.

Brown fat is the substance surrounding your organs and differs from white fat in many ways. Brown fat acts as a thermostat and helps the body acclimate to hot and cold temperatures. It aids in weight loss by helping the body convert calories into heat energy via thermogenesis. Brown fat helps burn 25 percent of all fat calories. In this regard, brown fat is an important element of metabolism.

As we age, brown fat begins to lose its burning capability. Think about the difference between senior citizens, who are often sensitive to the cold and gain weight in their later years, and youngsters, who are height-weight proportionate and tolerate cold temperatures very easily. Young children can be outside in cold temperatures wearing just t-shirts and shorts and not be cold because their brown fat is running in high gear.

How do you increase brown fat? **Gamma-linolenic Acid** (GLA), like its twin from the Omega 3 family (EPA and DHA), helps fight heart disease, cancer and arthritis and also promotes weight loss. GLA in your daily diet is the raw material needed by prostaglandins to stimulate brown fat. Dietary deficiencies and disease may block or slow the conversion of LA into GLA. This is one reason it may be necessary to find direct essential fatty acids that contain GLA. The highest sources of GLA are borage and evening primrose oil.

Health Concerns with Borage Oil

Borage oil is safe for most adults. Do not take borage oil if:

- You are pregnant or breast-feeding
- You have liver disease
- You have kidney disease
- You have schizophrenia

There is some concern that borage oil can increase the risk of bruising and bleeding when used with blood thinners. Before you start taking borage oil, talk with your health care professional.

Where Do You Find Omega 6 Fatty Acids?

Just as you must search for Omega 3 fatty acids, you must also search for healthy Omega 6 fatty acids. The best Omega 6 oils are unrefined and taste like the seeds from which they were mechanically pressed. Soybeans, soybean oil, sunflower seeds, sesame seeds, pumpkin seeds, pumpkin seed oil, flaxseed oil and leafy greens are excellent sources of Omega 6 fats. Safflower, sunflower, soybean and sesame oils can be good choices, but only if they are unrefined. You will find unrefined oils most often in health and natural food stores. Most raw nuts also contain some Omega 6 fatty acids. To get adequate amounts of GLA into your diet, choose unrefined borage or evening primrose oil. You must protect Omega 6 fatty acids, just like the Omega 3 fatty acids, by buying them fresh and storing them safely in the refrigerator or freezer. Remember, do not heat or cook with any Omega 3 or Omega 6 oils. Heat destroys the benefits of these oils. Use only monounsaturated fats such as extra virgin olive oil or expeller pressed canola oil for cooking.

Arachidonic Acid Overload

Unlike Omega 3 fatty acids, which are universally healthy fats, there are great differences in the quality and health benefits of Omega 6 fats. Arachidonic Acid (AA) is the end product of Omega 6 fatty acid conversions (LA→GLA→AA). The body needs some arachidonic acid to function optimally, but too much can promote certain diseases. Refined oils, such as soybean or corn oil along with meat, especially red meat, can lead to an arachidonic overload. To correct this, try to consume more unrefined oils and limit your consumption of red meat and refined oils. Omega 3 fats also help by blocking the conversion to arachidonic acid, keeping your essential fats in balance.

How Much Omega 6 Fat Should You Eat?

Make an effort to get one or two servings (1-2 tbs.) of unrefined, quality Omega 6s in your diet each day. Use unrefined oils, raw nuts, seeds or leafy greens in your daily diet.

Omega 3 and Omega 6 Fats in Balance

Your body functions best when your diet contains a balanced ratio of Omega 3 and Omega 6 fatty acids. In the United States, we currently eat an unbalanced ratio of Omega 3 and Omega 6 fatty acids. The World Health Organization recommends a two-to-one ratio of essential fatty acids: two Omega 6 fats to one Omega 3 fat. In the U.S., we have a sixteen-to-one (or greater) Omega 6 to Omega 3 ratio.

This imbalance may lead to heart disease, diabetes, cancer, obesity, arthritis, inflammation, Alzheimer's disease and a host of other auto-immune diseases. A large percentage of the American population over the age of 45 is regularly taking self-prescribed, over-the-counter anti-inflammatories such as aspirin and ibuprofen. These anti-inflammatories may address the symptoms but not the underlying causes, which may be due to an imbalance in the consumption of Omega 3 and Omega 6 fats. Consequently, many modern-day health problems can be relieved by bringing these fatty acids back into balance.

Since the 1960's, U.S. consumption of Omega 6 oils has doubled. One of the reasons the U.S. population is overeating Omega 6 fats is that they are in almost every refined or processed food we consume. Similar to the widespread use of trans-fatty acids, manufacturers use refined Omega 6 fatty acids such as corn oil and soybean oil. With technological improvements in oil extraction over the last sixty years, oil manufacturers can use inexpensive raw materials, such as corn or soybeans, from which to extract and refine a great deal of oil. The result? An excessive amount of low-quality, refined Omega 6 fats that are abundant in restaurants and grocery stores.

Tips for Improving the Quality of Fat in Your Diet

Don't become overwhelmed by trying to balance out your Omega 3 and 6 fats. Start with flaxseed oil or flaxmeal. Flaxseed oil and flaxmeal have both Omega 3 and Omega 6 fats and are from an unrefined source. Cold water fish also has both Omega 3 and Omega 6 fats. Try eating one or two servings per week.

There is no other nutrient available that can heal the body and keep it healthy from infancy to old age like good fats.

Recommended Fat Consumption Based on Daily Calorie Intake		
Total Calories	Grams of Fat	Number of Fat Calories
1,200	27-47	240-420
1,500	33-58	300-525
1,800	40-70	360-630
2,000	44-78	400-700
2,500	56-97	500-875
3,000	67-117	600-1050

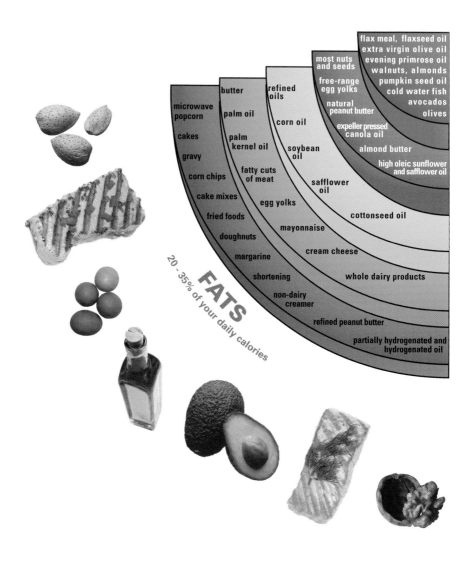

flax meal, flaxseed oil
extra virgin olive oil
evening primrose oil
walnuts, almonds
pumpkin seed oil
cold water fish
avocados
olives

most nuts and seeds

free-range egg yolks

natural peanut butter

expeller pressed canola oil

almond butter

high oleic sunflower and safflower oil

butter

refined oils

corn oil

microwave popcorn

palm oil

cakes

palm kernel oil

gravy

soybean oil

fatty cuts of meat

corn chips

safflower oil

cake mixes

egg yolks

fried foods

cottonseed oil

doughnuts

mayonnaise

margarine

cream cheese

shortening

whole dairy products

non-dairy creamer

refined peanut butter

partially hydrogenated and hydrogenated oil

FATS
20 - 35% of your daily calories

Reminder: Use the food target to guide your food choices.

Fat Summary Guide

TYPE	TRANS-FATS	SATURATED	MONO-UNSATURATED (Omega 9)	POLY-UNSATURATED (Omega 3)	POLY-UNSATURATED (Omega 6)
QUALITY/ SOURCE	**Poor:** margarine, shortening, cakes, pies, doughnuts, microwave popcorn, processed snacks, candy bars, partially hydrogenated oils, deep fried foods, many fast foods, most commercial baked goods, gravy, refined peanut butter, non-dairy creamer	**Better:** wild game, free-range eggs/ chicken, most raw nuts, lean meats, skim milk, soy milk, Feta, goat, Mozzarella cheeses **Poor:** tropical oils, butter, processed meats, whole milk, processed cheese, ice cream, red meat	**Best:** extra virgin olive oil, expeller pressed canola oil, almonds, almond oil, almond butter, avocados, avocado oil, olives, filberts, brazil nuts **Better:** natural peanut butter, pecans, cashews, pistachio nuts, high oleic sunflower and safflower oils	**Best:** ground flaxseeds, flaxseed oil, cold water fish (trout, salmon, tuna, mackerel), walnuts, walnut oil, leafy greens	**Best:** soybeans, soybean oil, sunflower seeds, sesame seeds, pumpkin seeds, pumpkin seed oil, borage oil, evening primrose oil, hemp oil, leafy greens
HEALTH BENEFITS:	**Detrimental to your health**		Wonderful health benefits when using unrefined sources	Wonderful health benefits when using unrefined sources	Wonderful health benefits when using unrefined sources
USES:	To enhance processed foods	To enhance taste and shelf life	Great for cooking, baking, salads, spreads	**DO NOT HEAT THESE FATS!** Use in salads, smoothies, cereal Store in refrigerator	
SERVING SIZE:	**Avoid these harmful fats (Bad Fats)** No acceptable levels	**Avoid them** <5% daily calories 1/2–1 tbs/day	10-15% daily calories 2-3 tbs/day	10% daily calories 1-2 tbs/day 1-2 servings of cold water fish/week (cooking does not harm fish fats) 1 tbs flaxseed oil or 2 tbs flaxmeal/100 lbs body weight	10% daily calories 1-2 tbs/day

Chapter 7

What Are We Drinking?

Desire creates the power.
– Raymond Holliwell

What *are* we drinking? Over the last thirty years, the variety of foods available, and the consumption of certain foods, has changed dramatically. The same is true of the types and quantity of beverages we drink. Soda pop is currently the number one beverage consumed in the United States. The average American drinks over seventy gallons of soda pop every year. This number continues to grow, especially among children and teenagers. Beer, coffee and milk run a distant second, at 25 to 30 gallons per person per year. On average, we each drink eight to ten gallons of fruit juices and tea per year. One piece of good news is that bottled water consumption is climbing, currently averaging over 20 gallons per person per year. The chart below shows trends in beverage consumption in the U.S. between 1970 and 2002, according to the Beverage Marketing Company, the leading research and consulting firm dedicated to the beverage industry.

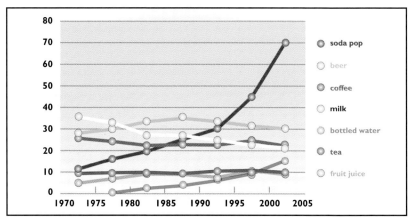

The most negative implication of the upward trend in soda pop and juice consumption is the corresponding increase in sugar consumption. On average, Americans each consume 182 pounds of sugar and over 25 pounds of artificial sweeteners each year. This increase corresponds to the upward trend in Type 2 diabetes, obesity and bone loss.

Splenda® and Stevia Plus™ to the Rescue

Healthier alternatives to artificial sweeteners are Splenda® and Stevia Plus™. Both have few or no calories and little impact on blood glucose levels.

Splenda contains dextrose, maltodextrin and sucralose and can be purchased in most grocery stores. Splenda is made from sugar, tastes just like sugar and may be used in your favorite recipe or beverage.

Stevia Plus contains fiber and is made from the stevia plant found in South America. Stevia Plus is low in calories, has little effect on blood glucose and is an excellent option for individuals with diabetes. Stevia Plus is sold as powder and liquid and can be found in most natural food stores. Like Splenda, Stevia can be used as a sweetener in your favorite recipes or beverages. Stevia Plus is a healthier, natural alternative to refined sugar or artificial sweeteners.

Gotta Have My Caffeine

Americans love the legal buzz they get from caffeine. The USDA reports that the average American consumes about 240 milligrams of caffeine daily, mostly from coffee. People crave caffeine because of the jump start it gives them.

Caffeine stimulates the adrenal glands which increases heart rate, blood pressure and alertness. With overuse, caffeine may cause sleep difficulties, jitters, anxiety and heartburn.

Caffeine also increases the acidity level of your blood. This leads to bone loss due to loss of calcium and magnesium. We are now seeing osteoporosis (low bone density) in women in their 20s and 30s due to high caffeine intake from soda pop and coffee.

Is caffeine addictive? There are many opinions about the addictive properties of caffeine. Mine is that it has some addictive properties. Often, people who eliminate caffeine experience headaches and irritability for a short time.

If you regularly find yourself tired, anxious and overly stressed, you may want to wean yourself from caffeine and replace your caffeinated beverages with —you guessed it— water. You will be amazed how good you feel when your body is fully hydrated.

Water–The Body's Drink of Choice

75 percent of the American population is chronically dehydrated.

Water is essential for keeping the body healthy. 70 percent of the body is water. Even a small drop in water consumption compromises the body in many ways. But do we truly understand the impact of inadequate water consumption?

Unintentional chronic dehydration may be the root of many serious diseases, including asthma, endocrine and kidney problems, high blood pressure and other cardiovascular diseases, arthritis, ulcers, pancreatitis, digestive difficulties, low back pain and obesity.

Water is the body's cleansing and waste removal fluid. It also aids in digestion and metabolism. Not having enough water contributes to fatigue. As the body becomes dehydrated, blood is the place your body looks for more water. When the body pulls water from the blood, blood volume decreases and energy (cardiac output) also decreases. Dehydration causes stress, and stress causes further dehydration.

You should drink 60 to 80 ounces (eight to ten glasses) of water every day. Do this by drinking ten ounces of water at every meal or snack and an additional 30 to 40 ounces throughout the day. Your body's need for water increases as you exercise more.

Let water be your drink of choice. Start replacing your current beverages (soda pop, coffee, fruit juice, alcohol) with water. Spice up your water with a slice of lemon, lime or orange.

> 66 I am so pleased with Chris's Meal Patterning program. Meal Patterning has not only lowered my cholesterol but also raised my HDL and lowered my overall cardiac risk. I have much energy, strength and stamina. The constant cravings and hungry feelings I had are gone and I am much more alert throughout the day. 99
>
> **-Bruce Mortimer, D.V.M.**

Chapter 8

Fiber

If the world is cold, make it your business to build fires.
— Horace Traubel

Fiber is necessary for optimal health. Fiber helps reduce the risk of certain cancers, lowers cholesterol, stabilizes blood glucose and promotes regularity. Fiber absorbs water as it moves through the digestive tract and adds bulk to feces. Fiber moves food quickly through the digestive system and enhances fat loss. Fiber also slows down insulin response; this is one reason that eating whole fruit does not raise your blood glucose as much as drinking fruit juice which has no fiber. The National Cancer Institute recommends an intake of 25 grams of fiber daily. Most Americans eat 15 grams of fiber per day.

Types of Fiber

1. Water-soluble: Water-soluble fiber helps reduce cholesterol and slows insulin response. Some water-soluble fiber sources are oatmeal, oat bran, barley, beans, peas and apples.

2. Water-insoluble: Water-insoluble fiber helps supply the bulk that keeps food moving quickly through the digestive tract, acting like a broom sweeping out undigested material, promoting regularity and reducing the risk of certain kinds of cancers. Leafy vegetables, whole grains, root vegetables and skins from fruits and vegetables all contain water-insoluble fiber.

We can easily obtain fiber by eating foods in their most natural state, such as whole grains, nuts, seeds, fruits and vegetables.

Tips for adding more fiber to your diet include

• Sneak in vegetables whenever you can. Don't over-cook as this decreases the fiber content.

• Eat more whole fruits. Berries, apples and dried fruits are high in fiber.

• Eat more beans. Beans are loaded with fiber. A half cup of beans contains four to six grams of fiber.

• Eat whole grains instead of refined white versions. Look for whole grain breads, pastas and cereals.

• Bring on the nuts and seeds. Raw walnuts, almonds, flaxseeds and flaxmeal are excellent sources of fiber.

Fiber Grams per Serving of Various Foods

garbanzo beans (1/2 cup)	8	kale (3 oz.)	3
flaxmeal (3 tbs.)	6	broccoli slaw (3 oz.)	3
whole grain bread (1 slice)	6	walnuts (1/4 cup)	3
broccoli (1 cup)	5	almonds (1/4 cup)	3
apple (1 apple)	4	spinach (3 oz.)	2
blueberries (3/4 cup)	4	raisins (1/4 cup)	2
raspberries (3/4 cup)	4	white bread (1 slice)	1
oatmeal (1/2 cup)	4	beef	0
potato (1 potato)	3	chicken	0
green beans (1 cup)	3	tuna	0

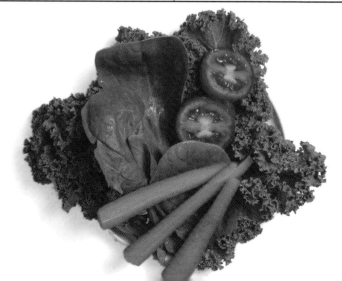

Chapter 9

Do You Have Healthy Bones?

What the mind can conceive and believe, it can achieve.
– Napoleon Hill

People want healthy bones but don't know how food affects bones. Calcium gets so much attention that many people believe having healthy bones depends only on getting enough calcium.

Americans have poor bone health compared to people in other countries. The current recommendation for calcium intake in the United States is 1,000 milligrams per day for ages 19–50 and 1,200 milligrams per day for ages 50 and over. The average American consumes 900-1,000 milligrams of calcium per day, yet osteoporosis affects 10 million American men and women, 300,000 of whom suffer hip fractures in a year. Approximately 50 percent of all women and 20 percent of all men over the age of 65 will experience bone fractures.

Countries such as Japan and Yugoslavia have a much lower intake of calcium, 300-600 mg per day, and a much lower incidence of osteoporosis. Countries with the highest average calcium intake—the United States, New Zealand and Sweden—have higher, not lower, hip fracture rates.

Calcium intake plays an important role for bone health, but other factors contribute to healthy bones.

What Weakens Bones?

1. **Lack of weight-bearing exercise:** Many people consider walking a weight-bearing exercise. Walking is a good form of exercise, but does little to stimulate the bones of the spine and upper body. This is one reason I recommend some form of strength training to almost everyone. If our bones are not adequately stressed, they begin to weaken as we age. Strength training increases bone density by placing added stress on the bones.

2. **Acidosis and Osteoporosis:** More and more, research links acidosis to osteoporosis. We now see low bone density (weak bones) in young women. Why is this happening? There is a direct link between acid-alkaline balance and bone health. Bone is sensitive to small changes in blood pH. As the body becomes more acidic, pH levels change with three bad results.

• Bone begins to break down. • Bone regeneration is inhibited.

• Bone mineral loss is increased.

What Makes the Body Acidic?

1. **Eating too much protein:** Getting more than 25 percent of your daily calories from protein may cause the body to become acidic. When proteins break down, they must be neutralized by buffering minerals. If your protein intake is too high, buffering minerals from bone may be depleted and a decrease in bone mass occurs.

2. **High dietary intake of phosphate/phosphoric acid:** Foods such as processed cheese, ice cream, artificial sweeteners, fried foods, beef, cocoa, sugar, table salt and cottage cheese create high acid levels in the blood. Beverages such as colas, coffee and beer also increase acid levels. The body must draw upon buffers to neutralize the excess acid. With the average American teenager consuming three to six cola beverages per day, you can see why osteoporosis is now seen in young women. Since men generally have greater bone density than women, the impact of phosphate and phosphoric acid on men's bone health is not as great.

3. **High levels of stress:** Stress can eat up our bones quickly. Stress triggers the hormones adrenaline and cortisol. Adrenaline and cortisol accelerate the acidity level of blood, leading to mineral loss.

4. **Inadequate amounts of calcium and magnesium:** Target intake for calcium is 1,000 milligrams per day for adults up to age 50 and 1,200 milligrams per day for those over age 50. The target for magnesium is 420 milligrams per day for men and 320 milligrams per day for women. Food sources high in calcium and magnesium include tofu, oatmeal, milk, figs, beans, spinach, leafy greens, soybeans, salmon, almonds, broccoli, squash and barley.

5. **Getting enough Vitamin D:** Vitamin D plays an important role in keeping your bones strong and healthy. Recommended intake for Vitamin D is 600-800 units per day. Very few foods naturally contain Vitamin D. Eat foods high in Vitamin D such as salmon, tuna, free-range eggs, fortified breakfast cereals and dairy products. Getting a few minutes of sunlight a day also increases Vitamin D production. Taking a multivitamin is an easy and sure way of getting enough Vitamin D daily.

What Can You Do to Keep Your Bones Healthy?

There are seven important tips for keeping your bones healthy. Try to incorporate all seven into your life to protect your skeleton for the duration of your long and healthy life.

1. **Start a total body strength training program.** Exercise twice a week for 15 to 30 minutes. See Chapter 20 to learn more about strength training.

2. **Eat more fruits and vegetables.** Most fruits and vegetables—especially fruits—have high alkaline levels and help maintain alkaline–acid balance.

3. **Eat high-calcium, high-magnesium foods.** Leafy green vegetables, low-fat dairy products, soy products, salmon, almonds, asparagus, broccoli, squash, figs, beans, oatmeal and barley are excellent sources.

4. **Get enough Vitamin D**. Eat foods such as salmon, tuna, free-range eggs, fortified breakfast cereals and dairy products. Taking a multivitamin is a sure way of getting enough Vitamin D per day.

5. **Avoid foods and beverages high in phosphates, phosphoric acid and caffeine.**

6. **Control your stress.** Some techniques to help your stress levels are positive self-talk, quiet time-out periods throughout the day, meditation, yoga, exercise, soft music, a cup of herbal tea or a brisk walk around the block.

7. **Drink plenty of water.**

Chapter 10

What Should
You Feed Your Kids?

We cannot direct the wind, but we can adjust the sails.
– Unknown

A question regularly asked during my Meal Patterning seminars is, "What should I feed my kids?" I have teen-aged twins of my own, Kristen and Matt. From my own experience, trying to get kids to eat in a healthy way can be challenging. I would like to share some of my own experiences trying to shape my kids' nutritional patterns.

When Kristen and Matt were still in high chairs, I thought it would be a good idea for them to eat a healthier type of macaroni and cheese. Dinner time can be a difficult time for parents of young children. Finding food the kids like that is healthy for them is hard. Kristen and Matt liked macaroni and cheese, so I decided to replace their usual macaroni and cheese with a healthy version (whole grain macaroni and soy cheese). I figured if they didn't see me prepare the different variety they wouldn't know the difference. Keep in mind this was 1987 and at that time many "health foods" didn't taste very good. When they first started to eat the macaroni and cheese, I was excited and smug, thinking my plan had worked. To my chagrin, both kids spit it out and started to cry after a few seconds of chewing. This was my first attempt at shaping their nutritional patterns and I had failed miserably. But I learned a valuable lesson—changes to meal patterns need to be developed slowly for your children, as well as for yourself.

With the explosion of refined foods, our kids are exposed to increasingly more unhealthy choices. Isn't it interesting that there is a tremendous rise in obesity, type 2 diabetes, poor bone health, allergies, attention deficit hyperactivity disorder (ADHD) and fatigue in our kids? How can we improve this?

One of the healthiest things you can do for your kids is to give them good fats, especially the essential fatty acid Omega 3. When my kids were younger, my wife and I would sneak good fats into their diets so they have been eating good fats such as walnuts, almonds, cold water fish, extra virgin olive oil and, of course, flaxmeal and flaxseed oil regularly. But as they entered high school, I felt it was time they started making some of these choices on their own and taking more responsibility for their own eating patterns. After all, they'd heard my sermons and lectures about the benefits of good fats.

When left to their own devices though, it was clear I hadn't gotten through to them. Nutrition isn't necessarily a high priority for teenagers. They would eat good fats occasionally, but not regularly. I knew I couldn't be the "food police" forever. I needed to understand what was important to them and to accept reality. It was time to be creative. I needed to find some way to show them how eating the right foods could help them in the areas that were important to them.

Boys and girls have different eating patterns and often look at food differently, especially as they get older. Girls are much more concerned about their bodies and appearance, and their eating patterns are influenced by magazines, television, movies and family. Perhaps the strongest influence is their friends and schoolmates. When Kristen was in middle school, I noticed that she was tired and irritable when she came home from school. She had lost the pep in her step. After she ate, she started to perk up. I discovered—by asking many questions—that Kristen's meal patterns were the problem. She started her day with cold cereal and skim milk for breakfast. At lunch she was eating one salt bagel and a bottle of water. After school, she was usually engaged in some kind of extracurricular activity. By the time Kristen walked in the door at 6:00 p.m., she had consumed only 200 calories of refined carbohydrates, little fat, and only a trace amount of protein over an eleven-hour day.

A growing, active, teen-aged girl needs much more from her nutritional plan than Kristen was getting. To stay healthy and perform optimally, Kristen had to change her meal patterns. She began by eating more frequently throughout the day, adding more calories to her daily intake. She also began to look at the quality of foods she was eating, deciding to pack her lunch so she could eat what she wanted and not be limited by the school menu. She also packed an after-school snack. The foods she chose weren't perfect but she made great improvements to her nutritional plan. She developed a plan she liked and could manage, and her energy and pep returned.

For my son, Matt, it's the game of golf. Matt lives, eats and breathes golf and plays on his high school golf team. During his sophomore year, I casually reminded him that one of the benefits of consuming flaxseed oil, high in Omega 3s, was that it might help him concentrate, relax and have better focus. I suggested that improved concentration, relaxation and focus might help his golf game, and benefit him in the classroom. He tried it and has been regularly taking 1-½ tablespoons of flaxseed oil daily before school. He just takes it straight and washes it down with orange juice. He believes it has helped his golf game and I believe it has helped him in the classroom, not to mention providing him with all the other health benefits associated with a more balanced diet.

As parents, we want the best for our kids—we want them to develop into healthy, happy adults. When it comes to nutritional patterns, parents must set the tone. Healthy nutritional patterns take time and energy to develop, and require compromise and negotiation along the way.

Start by slowly cleaning out the refined foods in your house. Replace them with natural and less refined food items. For example,

Current food item	Better choice
refined peanut butter	natural peanut butter
mayonnaise	canola mayonnaise
soda pop	water
French fries	make your own by baking with extra virgin olive oil
sugared cereals	less refined cereals with added fruit
chips/crackers	snack foods with higher quality fats
white bread	whole grain bread
candy bars	energy bars
fruit juice	whole fruit

Kid Tips

• **Set the tone.** Practice healthy nutritional patterns yourself. Your kids will follow your lead.

• **Make one small change per week.** Slowly replace unhealthy food choices and patterns.

• **Place the food target on the refrigerator.** Refer to the food target on a daily basis. Educate your kids about quality food choices from the food target.

• **What's for dinner?** You don't have to become a short order cook to keep everyone happy. Develop healthy mealtime patterns and stick to your guns.

• **Have healthy snacks available.** Have easy, accessible snacks around the house such as nuts, fresh fruit, low-fat dairy products, yogurt, string cheese and cold cereals. Make your own smoothie drinks for after-school snacks and for before or after sporting activities.

• **Bring on the fat.** Have your kids eat quality fats every day.

These are just a few ideas to get you started. As your kids grow and mature, so will their meal patterns. Educate them, be patient and lead by example. Help them recognize the benefits of eating well. And don't worry when they say, "There's nothing to eat in this house!" They won't starve.

Section 2

Steps to Success

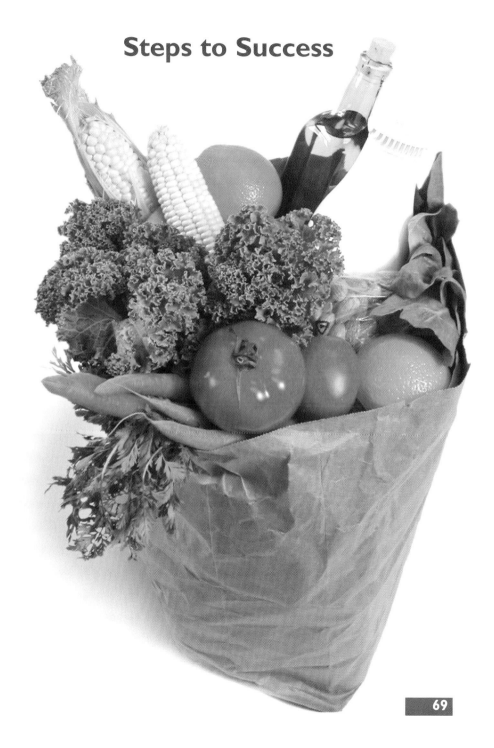

Let the Journey Begin

It is great to have an end to journey towards,
but it is the journey that matters, in the end.

– Ursula Le Guin

Now that you have come this far, you have the knowledge to succeed. In the following chapters, I lay out steps to help you succeed in your journey to healthier eating. Begin this journey at your own pace. Research shows that small changes are more successful than multiple behavior changes all at once. Baby steps are the key; otherwise, it can be overwhelming. If you want to start with one small change or to make multiple changes, it's up to you. Meal Patterning is about educating and motivating you to invest in healthy eating. One small step leads to the next step, which leads to more. Take the first step and don't look back. Invest in yourself. You're worth it.

Steps Toward a Successful Journey

- **Set realistic goals.**
- **Be specific.**
- **Have a plan of action—your road map.**
- **Get support from family and friends.**
- **Keep a record of how you are doing.**
- **Prepare yourself for roadblocks along the way.**

Chapter 11

Step 1
Develop a Road Map–Set Your Goals

> All I know is that the first step is to create the vision there—
> the beautiful vision that creates the want power.
>
> – Arnold Schwarzenegger

"Am I ready for a change?" This is the first question you must ask yourself on your journey toward a change in behavior. Answer honestly. You must first determine your goals and get a clear picture of where you want to go and what you want from your nutritional plan. What is the vision you have of yourself? What do you want to change? Do you want more energy? Do you want to improve your fitness level? Do you want to wear a smaller dress or pair of slacks? Do you want to improve your health by lowering your blood pressure or cholesterol?

Think seriously about what you want to change and why. Be as specific as possible about what you want and why you want it. Empower yourself. Set your goals, write them down and look at them daily. Only you know what will work for you. You can accomplish your goals, but you must first know where you are going.

Don't wait. Act now. Tomorrows turn into lifetimes.

---

66 My motto is "age is only a number" and with that attitude I have maintained my physical activities at a very high level throughout my life. However, my physical appearance and my performance were two different things. When I looked in the mirror, I was not happy with my physique. I was impressed with my brother's and his clients' results, so I went to him for advice. Chris recommended that I sign up for the over-age-40 Masters Bodybuilding contest with him. The problem for me was changing my eating habits. So, with the help of Chris and Tab Jackson, Michigan Athletic Club personal trainer, my journey began.

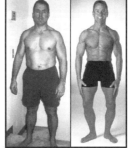

Over the next 12 weeks I learned to eat clean—first, cutting all refined foods and learning to eat good fats. At the end of that 12 weeks I lost 36 pounds and went from 22.5 percent body fat to 7 percent and won my first Grand Rapids Western Michigan Masters Bodybuilding Championship. I noticed that by eating healthier, I have a great deal more energy. Not only did good nutrition help me reach my weight goal, but my sleeping habits, work and athletic performance have all improved. Nutrition was the key to improving all aspects of my life and I feel younger than ever. 99

- Nick Johnson, age 48

Chapter 12

Step 2
Keep a Daily Meal Patterning Food Log

Joy comes from using your potential.
– Will Schultz

Monitor your daily eating, drinking, activity and sleeping habits and record them in a daily food log. Use the food log to create awareness of where you are and changes you want to make. Analyze your daily food log and notice patterns that sabotage your goals. Do you skip meals and load up on calories at the end of the day? Do you eat too much food at one sitting? Do you eat too many carbohydrates, not enough protein, the wrong types of fats? Do you eat when you are hungry, or when you are bored, upset or anxious? The daily food log gives you a place to start.

How to Use the Daily Food Log

Write the time of each meal. Under description, write what you ate and approximate serving sizes. Place a check inside the food target to represent a carbohydrate, protein or fat. Many foods you choose will be a combination of all three macronutrients. Remember that the most nutritious foods are closer to the center of the target. At the bottom of the daily food log, indicate the amount of water you drank, hours you slept and kinds of physical activities you performed, then write a brief description of your thoughts, feelings and energy level during the day. The daily food log is a learning tool that you can use over and over.

As you begin your Meal Patterning journey, you need to learn more about grocery shopping. This will help you find foods you enjoy and make good decisions about the foods you purchase.

Translating food labels for healthy shopping does not take a calculator or a great deal of time. Learning how to read food labels quickly and accurately is easy and will help you see through marketing gimmicks. Once you understand the content of foods, you can make good decisions about what to eat, meal planning and tweaking your favorite recipes.

Sample Food Log

DAILY FOOD LOG - Day: _Saturday_ **Date:** _4/19/03_

Meal	Description	Target
Breakfast Time: _6:30_	Oatmeal sliced strawberries soy milk walnuts	(carbohydrates/fats/proteins target diagram)
Snack 1 Time: _10:00_	CJ's Smoothie water flaxseed oil whey protein powder banana frozen berries	(carbohydrates/fats/proteins target diagram)
Lunch Time: _12:00_	Big Salad spinach and Romaine lettuce walnuts & raisins tuna in water balsamic vinegar & extra virgin olive oil	(carbohydrates/fats/proteins target diagram)
Snack 2 Time: _2:45_	Low-fat cottage cheese Pineapple Slivered almonds	(carbohydrates/fats/proteins target diagram)
Dinner Time: _6:00_	Salmon Fillet Redskin potatoes Kale, onion, garlic, extra virgin olive oil	(carbohydrates/fats/proteins target diagram)
Snack 3 Time: _9:30_	Green Apple Natural peanut butter	(carbohydrates/fats/proteins target diagram)

Water (8oz)	☑ ☑ ☑ ☑ ☑ ☑ ☑ ☑ ☐ ☐
Sleep (hours)	4 ☐ 5 ☐ 6 ☐ 7 ☐ 8 ☑ 9 ☐ 10 ☐
Activity / Exercise	☑ Cardio ☑ Strength ☑ Flexibility ☐ Other
Comments	Great day! Energy was high, sleep was restful.

Chapter 13

Step 3
Translate Food Labels for Healthy Shopping

When we know what we want,
we can think and speak positively with great expectations.
— Iyanla Vanzant

Understanding Food Labels

1. **How long is the ingredient list?** Generally, the shorter the ingredient list, the fewer refinements have been made to the food. You won't see an ingredient list on fresh fruits and vegetables. These products are in their natural state. Choose quality ingredients and a short ingredient list.

Let's compare two breakfast cereals, oatmeal and Blueberry Crisp™. The oatmeal has only one ingredient, rolled oats. It is high in fiber, has a better balance of carbohydrates, protein and fat, has no added bad fats or artificial ingredients, will maintain a steady blood glucose level and is very inexpensive. Contrast this with the Blueberry Crisp cereal, which has a very long ingredient list. It is high in sugar which will cause a greater swing in your blood glucose, contains trans-fatty acids and artificial flavors and is more expensive.

Oatmeal
INGREDIENTS: ROLLED OATS

Blueberry Crisp Cereal

INGREDIENTS: CORN, SUGAR, BLUEBERRIES (BLUEBERRIES, HIGH FRUCTOSE CORN SYRUP, GLYCEROL, SAFFLOWER OIL, CITRIC ACID, CALCIUM LACTATE, POTASSIUM SORBATE [PRESERVATIVE], NATURAL BLUEBERRY FLAVORING), ROLLED OATS, SLICED ALMONDS, PARTIALLY HYDROGENATED SOYBEAN AND/OR COTTONSEED OIL, SALT, HONEY, MALT EXTRACT, RICE, PARTIALLY HYDROGENATED SUNFLOWER OIL, HIGH FRUCTOSE CORN SYRUP, NATURAL AND ARTIFICIAL FLAVOR, NONFAT MILK, MOLASSES, CORN SYRUP
VITAMINS AND MINERALS: SODIUM ASCORBATE AND ASCORBIC ACID, NIACINAMIDE, FERRIC ORTHOPHOSPHATE, PYRIDOXINE HYDROCHLORIDE, VITAMIN A PALMITATE, RIBOFLAVIN, THIAMIN HYDROCHLORIDE, FOLIC ACID, VITAMIN D.

2. The ingredient list starts with the most predominant ingredient and continues in descending order.

In the next example, we compare two types of Ranch salad dressing. Ranch dressing A has a much shorter ingredient list and a higher quality of fat (expeller pressed canola oil) with no added preservatives. Ranch dressing B has a longer ingredient list, has a poor quality fat listed as its first ingredient (soybean oil) and also contains an unhealthy food additive, monosodium glutamate (MSG). Once you understand the labels, choosing dressing A is easy.

A

Natural Dressing

INGREDIENTS: EXPELLER PRESSED CANOLA OIL, WATER, CIDER VINEGAR, BUTTERMILK POWDER, ORGANIC SUGAR, SEA SALT, EGG POWDER, ONION POWDER, GARLIC POWDER, XANTHAM GUM.

B

Refined Dressing

INGREDIENTS: SOYBEAN OIL, WATER, VINEGAR, SUGAR, EGG YOLKS, SALT, CONTAINS LESS THAN 2% OF WHEY, ONIONS*, BUTTERMILK, MONOSODIUM GLUTAMATE, XANTHAM GUM, PHOSPHORIC ACID, WITH SORBIC ACID AND CALCIUM DISODIUM EDTA AS PRESERVATIVES, GARLIC*, POLYSORBATE 60, PARSLEY*, SPICE, NATURAL FLAVOR
*DRIED

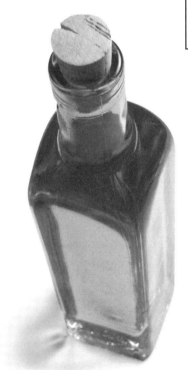

3. What is the serving size? When looking at any label, always check the serving size or number of servings in the product. Be aware that calories can add up quickly if your serving size exceeds the label recommendation.

Also be aware that manufacturers can label products low-fat, light or fat-free based on a serving size. If a product has less than .5 grams of fat, the Food and Drug Administration (FDA) will allow a product to be labeled fat-free, even if the product is 100 percent fat. For example, extra virgin olive oil C is 100 percent fat with 14 grams of fat per tablespoon. Compare that to the same brand of extra virgin olive oil no-stick cooking spray D which claims to be free of fat, calories and cholesterol. This labeling is based on less than .5 grams of fat per serving. In this example, a serving size of the no-stick spray is one-third of a second spray or less. I have tried this many times, and have found it impossible to spray the pan for only a third of a second. So, if you use the spray for a third of a second or less it is labeled fat-free, but what if you use it for a full three seconds? Read the labels and note the serving size.

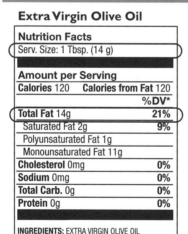

C

Extra Virgin Olive Oil

Nutrition Facts

Serv. Size: 1 Tbsp. (14 g)

Amount per Serving

		%DV*
Calories 120	Calories from Fat 120	
Total Fat 14g		**21%**
Saturated Fat 2g		9%
Polyunsaturated Fat 1g		
Monounsaturated Fat 11g		
Cholesterol 0mg		**0%**
Sodium 0mg		**0%**
Total Carb. 0g		**0%**
Protein 0g		**0%**

INGREDIENTS: EXTRA VIRGIN OLIVE OIL

D

Extra Virgin Olive Oil No StickSpray

Nutrition Facts

Serv. Size: 1/3 Second Spray (.266 g)

Amount per Serving

		%DV*
Calories 0	Calories from Fat 0	
Total Fat 0g		**0%**
Saturated Fat 0g		0%
Cholesterol 0mg		**0%**
Sodium 0mg		**0%**
Total Carb. 0g		**0%**
Protein 0g		**0%**

INGREDIENTS: 100% IMPORTED OLIVE OIL, GRAIN ALCOHOL FROM CORN (ADDED FOR CLARITY), LECITHIN FROM SOYBEANS (PREVENTS STICKING), AND PROPELLENT.

4. What kind of fat? It is important to learn how to distinguish healthy, good fats from unhealthy, bad fats with the goal of eliminating trans-fatty acids from your diet. Trans-fatty acids are in any product that lists hydrogenated or partially hydrogenated oils. The FDA will soon require that food labels include the amount of trans-fatty acids in products. Try to eliminate fractionated oils and cut back on saturated fats as well. Search for healthy, good fats such as monounsaturated fats and polyunsaturated (Omega 3 and unrefined Omega 6) fats.

A. Trans-fatty Acids

Margarine Spread

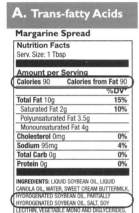

Nutrition Facts
Serv. Size: 1 Tbsp

Amount per Serving	
Calories 90	Calories from Fat 90
	%DV*
Total Fat 10g	15%
Saturated Fat 2g	10%
Polyunsaturated Fat 3.5g	
Monounsaturated Fat 4g	
Cholesterol 0mg	0%
Sodium 95mg	4%
Total Carb 0g	0%
Protein 0g	0%

INGREDIENTS: LIQUID SOYBEAN OIL, LIQUID CANOLA OIL, WATER, SWEET CREAM BUTTERMILK, HYDROGENATED SOYBEAN OIL, PARTIALLY HYDROGENATED SOYBEAN OIL, SALT, SOY LECITHIN, VEGETABLE MONO AND DIGLYCERIDES, (POTASSIUM SORBATE, SODIUM BENZOATE) AS PRESERVATIVES, ARTIFICIAL FLAVOR, VITAMIN A (PALMITATE), COLORED WITH BETA CAROTENE.

B. Saturated Fat

Whole Milk

Nutrition Facts
Serv. Size: 1 Cup

Amount per Serving	
Calories 150	Calories from Fat 70
	%DV*
Total Fat 8g	12%
Saturated Fat 5g	25%
Cholesterol 35mg	11%
Sodium 125mg	5%
Potassium 400mg	11%
Total Carb. 12g	4%
Dietary Fiber 0g	0%
Sugars 12g	25%
Protein 8g	16%

INGREDIENTS: Milk, Vitamin D₃

C. Fractionated Oil

Protein Bar

Nutrition Facts
Serv. Size: 1 Bar (75 g)

Amount per Serving	
Calories 260	Calories from Fat 60
	%DV*
Total Fat 6g	10%
Saturated Fat 3.5g	18%
Cholesterol 30mg	9%
Sodium 130mg	6%
Potassium 115mg	3%
Total Carb 9g	3%
Dietary Fiber <1g	3%
Sugars 5g	
Protein 30g	60%

INGREDIENTS: WHEY PROTEIN BLEND (WHEY PROTEIN CONCENTRATE, HYDROLYZED WHEY PROTEIN AND WHEY PROTEIN ISOLATE, CHOCOLATE COATING (POLYDEXTROSE, FRACTIONATED PALM KERNAL OIL, NON-FAT DRY MILK SOLIDS, COCOA POWDER, SOYA LECITHIN (AN EMULSIFIER), SALT, NATURAL FLAVOR AND SUCRALOSE), GLYCERINE, GELATIN, STRAWBERRY PASTE (STRAWBERRIES, SUGAR, DEXTROSE, CITRIC ACID, ARTIFICIAL FLAVORS, PECTIN, SODIUM CITRATE, AND SODIUM BENZOATE), SOY PROTEIN ISOLATE, WATER, RASPBERRY PASTE (CORN SYRUP, RED RASPBERRY PUREE, DEXTROSE, CELLULOSE GUM, CITRIC ACID, ARTIFICIAL FLAVORS, PECTIN, SODIUM CITRATE, AND SODIUM BENZOATE), PEANUT BUTTER, PEANUT FLOUR, RICE FLOUR, NATURAL AND ARTIFICIAL FLAVORS, CITRIC ACID, ZINMAG-6 (MAGNESIUM ASPARTATE, ZINC OXIDE, ZINC ASPARTATE, PYRIDOXINE, ZINC MONOMETHIONINE), POTASSIUM SORBATE, SUCRALOSE, MAY CONTAIN TRACES OF PEANUTS.

D. Monounsaturated Fat

Extra Virgin Olive Oil

Nutrition Facts
Serv. Size: 1 Tbsp. (14 g)

Amount per Serving	
Calories 120	Calories from Fat 120
	%DV*
Total Fat 14g	21%
Saturated Fat 2g	9%
Polyunsaturated Fat 1g	
Monounsaturated Fat 11g	
Cholesterol 0mg	0%
Sodium 0mg	0%
Total Carb. 0g	0%
Protein 0g	0%

INGREDIENTS: EXTRA VIRGIN OLIVE OIL

E. Polyunsaturated Fat (Omega 3)

Flaxseed Oil

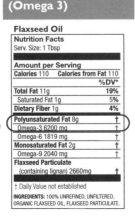

Nutrition Facts
Serv. Size: 1 Tbsp

Amount per Serving	
Calories 110	Calories from Fat 110
	%DV*
Total Fat 11g	19%
Saturated Fat 1g	5%
Dietary Fiber 1g	4%
Polyunsaturated Fat 8g	†
Omega-3 6200 mg	†
Omega-6 1819 mg	†
Monosaturated Fat 2g	†
Omega-9 2040 mg	†
Flaxseed Particulate (containing lignan) 2660mg	†

† Daily Value not established
INGREDIENTS: 100% UNREFINED, UNFILTERED, ORGANIC FLAXSEED OIL, FLAXSEED PARTICULATE.

F. Polyunsaturated Fat (Omega 6)

Borage Oil softgels

Nutrition Facts
Serv. Size: 1 Softgel

Amount per Serving	
Calories 10	Calories from Fat 10
	%DV*
Total Fat 1g	2%
Saturated Fat 0g	0%
Polyunsaturated Fat 1g	†
Monosaturated Fat 0g	†
Gamma Linolenic Acid (GLA)...1g	†
Linolenic Acid..................240 mg	†
Oleic Acid......................400 mg	†
Palmitic Acid..................200 mg	†
Stearic Acid....................60 mg	†

† Daily Value not established
INGREDIENTS: Borage Oil, Gelatin, Glycerin and Water.

5. What is the Carbohydrate/Protein/Fat ratio?

First determine the number of grams of the nutrient you are calculating.

Second, multiply the number of grams by the number of calories per gram. This will equal the calorie content of that nutrient in the product.

Third, divide the calories of that nutrient by the total calories in the product per serving, which will equal the percent of that nutrient in the product.

Calories per gram	
1 gram of fat = 9 calories	1 gram of protein = 4 calories
1 gram of carbohydrate = 4 calories	1 gram of alcohol = 7 calories

Example: Raisin Bagel

Use the final calculation to determine the proportion of each of the macronutrients within the total calories:

Step 1	Total Calories = 230 Total FAT = 2.5 grams Total CHO = 44 grams Total PRO = 8 grams
Step 2	2.5 grams x 9 calories = 22.5 calories from FAT 44 grams x 4 calories = 176 calories from CHO 8 grams x 4 calories = 32 calories from PRO
Step 3	22.5 FAT calories ÷ 230 total calories = 10% FAT 176 CHO calories ÷ 230 total calories = 77% CHO 32 PRO calories ÷ 230 total calories = 14% PRO

6. **Organic foods.** You may want to buy foods that are pesticide-free and grown in soil not fertilized with chemicals. Look for products labeled 100 percent organic.

Meal Patterning Shopping List

When you fill your shopping cart wisely, you are well on your way to a healthier nutritional program. If you have unhealthy food in your house, clean out the pantry and refrigerator so you can start fresh. Almost all of the food items you need can be purchased in conventional grocery stores. Many have a natural foods section. You may also want to find a natural foods store in your area. Most have a large selection of natural food items and a knowledgeable staff.

Below is a suggested shopping list. I have listed many items but this is by no means complete. Experiment and ask questions. Remember that shopping is a learning process, too, and can be fun. Go with a plan of action—make a list.

Fresh Vegetables
onions
redskin potatoes
yams
squash
zucchini
broccoli
cauliflower
celery
tomatoes
green/red/yellow peppers
carrots
Romaine lettuce
kale
collard greens
asparagus
mushrooms
spinach
garlic
cucumbers
cabbage slaw
broccoli slaw

Fresh Fruit
oranges
apples
grapes
peaches
cantaloupe
bananas
raisins
dates
figs
avocados
grapefruit
red raspberries
strawberries
blueberries
blackberries
watermelon
mango
apricots
sweet cherries
papaya
lemons

Meat/Poultry/Fish
boneless chicken breast
ground turkey
turkey breast
pork, lean
flank steak
beef tenderloin
fresh fish (salmon, tuna,
    trout, halibut, orange
    roughy)
canned salmon in water
canned tuna in water

Condiments
low-sodium chicken
    broth
Dijon mustard
salsa
Worcestershire sauce
Bragg's Liquid Aminos
balsamic vinegar
red wine vinegar

Seasonings
cumin
salt
pepper
thyme
oregano
basil
rosemary
chili powder
cilantro
vanilla
cinnamon
dill
garlic powder
dried mustard
almond extract
paprika

Frozen Vegetables
peas
green beans
spinach
mixed vegetables
stir-fry vegetables

Frozen Fruit
blueberries
strawberries
cherries
peaches
mixed fruit

**Cereals/Grains/
    Legumes**
rye bread
whole grain bread
peas
lentils
soybeans
black beans
Great Northern beans
garbanzo beans
extra-firm tofu
whole grain rice
whole grain pasta
whole grain tortillas
rolled oats
cold cereals

Juices
unsweetened cranberry
    juice
orange juice
grapefruit juice
low-sodium tomato juice

Eggs & Dairy
free-range eggs
low-fat cottage cheese
non-fat yogurt
low-fat Mozzarella
    cheese
Feta cheese
skim milk

Miscellaneous
bottled water
soy milk
pasta sauce
walnuts
almonds
fruit spread

crushed pineapple
natural applesauce
extra virgin olive oil
expeller pressed canola oil

Natural Foods Store
flaxseeds
flaxseed oil
borage oil
evening primrose oil
pumpkin seed oil
avocado oil
almond oil
walnut oil
wheat-free bread
rice bread
almond milk
oat milk
cold cereals
cooked cereals
waffles
chips
crackers
pizza
organic fruits
    & vegetables
Stevia Plus™
    (sugar substitute)
soy protein powder
whey protein powder
free-range eggs
organic chicken
buffalo
ostrich
salad dressings
almond butter
natural peanut butter
canola mayonnaise
nuts and seeds
green tea

Chapter 14

Step 4

Increase the Frequency of Your Meals

> Those who bring sunshine to the lives of others
> cannot keep it from themselves.
>
> – James Barrie

Spread Your Calories Throughout the Day

The first thing most people do when they want to lose weight is cut calories. They think the easiest way to cut calories is to skip meals. Unfortunately, you slow down your metabolism by skipping meals. Along with a slow metabolism, skipping meals alerts the body to release more of the fat-storing enzyme lipoprotein lipase. Remember—skipping meals is a strategy used by the Sumos to gain weight.

If one of your goals is revving up your metabolism, increase the frequency of your meals and spread your calories throughout the day. By eating more frequently, you will:

> • Increase your metabolic rate, allowing you to burn more calories;
>
> • Improve energy by maintaining a steadier blood glucose level;
>
> • Make better food choices because you won't be as hungry; and
>
> • Control portion sizes more easily.

During the first few weeks, make small changes. Eat the same foods and quantities, but eat more frequently. Instead of 2,000 calories in three meals each day, try eating the same number of calories split into four meals. After you have adjusted to four meals, try eating three meals and two snacks. Always eat breakfast. It is important to break your overnight fast and get your body running again for the day. **By eating more frequently and spacing out your calories evenly over the course of the day, you increase your metabolic rate and keep your blood glucose level steady.**

The chart below shows a comparison of how meals can be spaced throughout the day, with a progression from a poor plan to an ideal plan.

Poor 2000 calories		Good 2000 calories		Better 2000 calories		Best 2000 calories	
6:30 a.m.	Skip	6:30 a.m.	400 calories	6:30 a.m.	350 calories	6:30 a.m.	350 calories
Noon	Skip	Noon	700 calories	9:30 a.m.	250 calories	9:30 a.m.	250 calories
7:00 p.m	2000 calories	7:00 p.m.	900 calories	Noon	500 calories	Noon	450 calories
				3:30 p.m.	250 calories	3:00 p.m.	200 calories
				7:00 p.m.	650 calories	6:00 p.m.	600 calories
						8:00 p.m.	150 calories
1 meal		3 meals		3 meals, 2 snacks		3 meals, 3 snacks	

There will be days when you will find it difficult to eat frequently. Plan ahead and remember that enjoying fresh fruit and a few nuts, or a smoothie drink, is an easy and healthy way to improve your frequency of eating.

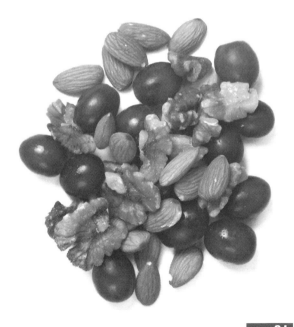

Chapter 15

Step 5
Quantity–How Much Are You Eating?

Everything is always impossible before it works.
– Hunt Greene

We can eat the right kinds of foods, correctly balanced, but if we eat too much at any one time (gorging), or over the course of the day, week, month or year, one or more of these problems may arise.

• over-production of insulin	• increased body fat
• imbalance of hormones	• poor health

How Many Calories Should You Eat Each Day?

The number of calories you need to eat per day depends on activity level, lean muscle mass, stress, frequency of meals and food quality.

Activity level: How much exercise do you get each day? How sedentary is your lifestyle? Is your job physical? How active is your day? Do you routinely walk, climb stairs or lift?

Lean muscle mass: The more lean muscle mass you have, the more calories your body burns at rest and throughout the day. This is why strength training is critical to maintaining or increasing your muscle.

Stress: Don't underestimate the role of stress and its effect on how many calories you need. Stress is vital for keeping us at the top of our game, but too much stress can lead to overeating—and the release of the hormone cortisol may lead to an increase in body fat.

Frequency of meals: When you eat more frequently, your body uses the food more efficiently, making it more difficult to overeat.

Food quality: Good carbohydrates, proteins and fats keep the body running at peak efficiency.

Your daily calorie needs may vary, depending on how your day unfolds. Try to listen to your body and its nutritional needs. If you are truly hungry, eat. But challenge yourself first—are you truly hungry, or just bored or stressed and looking for some relief? It will take time to develop new eating patterns. I have given you, below, a range of calories to consume throughout the day. Remember, this is just a range to work with. Your goal is not to count calories, but you must be conscious of the quantity of food you eat and this gives you a starting point.

Your body needs quality food in adequate amounts in order to stay healthy and to achieve optimal performance. You may exceed the high-end calorie range based on your activity level, lean muscle tissue, stress level, frequency and quality of meals.

Calorie Ranges per Day	
adult females	1,200-2,100
adult males	1,500-2,500

How Many Calories Should You Eat at Each Meal?

This may vary depending on the time of day, the last time you ate, or when you will eat next. Your goal is to spread your calories over the course of the day, with breakfast, lunch and dinner comprising your larger meals, and inserting small snacks in between. Eating more than 600 to 800 calories per meal, depending on your nutritional needs, may be too many calories at one meal. Eating high calorie meals will lead to high insulin levels, increased fat storage and unbalanced hormone levels.

Calories per Meal over the Course of a Day			
	1,200 calories	1,800 calories	2,500 calories
breakfast	250 calories	325 calories	450 calories
snack	100 calories	150 calories	250 calories
lunch	350 calories	500 calories	650 calories
snack	100 calories	150 calories	250 calories
dinner	400 calories	550 calories	700 calories
snack		125 calories	200 calories
Total	1,200 calories	1,800 calories	2,500 calories

Understanding Serving Sizes

The best laid plans for healthy eating can be negated if you are unaware of how much you are eating. A few years back, while monitoring my own nutritional program, I had exactly this problem. I was eating high-quality foods spread over the course of the day, but was not as lean as I wanted or expected to be. So, for three days, I filled out a food log, analyzed my meal plans and converted each meal and snack into specific calorie counts. I was shocked at my overall calorie intake, especially at breakfast. I took steps to reduce the calorie count, while maintaining the variety of foods.

For example, in my new version of breakfast, everything is essentially the same except the total calories are cut almost in half. The same benefits of the healthy breakfast are in place—quality carbohydrates, protein and fats—just in smaller amounts. I sometimes substitute one tablespoon of flaxseed oil for the walnuts, or three egg whites and one yolk for the protein powder.

By the way, this oatmeal recipe is not cooked and is served cold. I place all the ingredients in a small plastic bowl in the refrigerator overnight. The milk soaks in, the flavors mix, and in the morning I have a great-tasting, healthy breakfast (Oatmeal on the Run recipe—page 164).

Old Breakfast			Improved Breakfast	
oatmeal	1-1/2 cups	450 calories	2/3 cup	200 calories
walnuts	2 tbs.	240 calories	1 tbs.	120 calories
raisins	1/8 cup	65 calories	handful	40 calories
soy milk	10 oz.	120 calories	6 oz.	80 calories
protein powder	1 scoop	70 calories	1/2 scoop	35 calories
Total		**945 calories**		**475 calories**

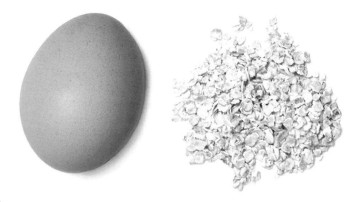

Quick Pick Food List

To speed up the process of understanding serving sizes, the Quick Pick Food List will help you create a serving size image. This will allow you to look at a food item and estimate the serving size and its approximate calories.

CHO (Carbohydrates)

Vegetables
1 cup = 8-15 grams = 32-60 calories
asparagus
mushrooms
zucchini
cucumbers
green, red, yellow peppers
Brussels sprouts
green beans
broccoli
spinach
kale
cabbage
onions
Romaine lettuce
peas (1/2 cup)
carrots (1/2 cup)
corn (1/2 cup)
potato (1 medium = 20 grams of CHO = 80 calories)
yam (1 medium = 20 grams of CHO = 80 calories)

Fruits
20 grams = 80 calories
apple (1 medium)
grapefruit (1 medium)
nectarine (1 large)
peach (1 large)
apricot (4 fresh)
dates (4 pitted)
green grapes (3/4 cup)
sweet cherries (3/4 cup fresh)
blackberries (1 cup)
cantaloupe (1-1/2 cups)
red raspberries (1-1/2 cups)
strawberries (1-1/2 cups)
watermelon (1-3/4 cups)
banana (1 small= 25 grams of CHO = 100 calories)
kiwi (2 = 25 grams of CHO = 100 calories)

Cereals, Grains, Legumes
30 grams = 120 calories
black beans (1/2 cup)
garbanzo beans (1/2 cup)
lentils (1/2 cup cooked)
bagel (1/2)
cooked cereal (1/2 cup)
cold cereal (1/2 to 1 cup)
flour tortilla (1)
pita bread (1-1/2 slices)
whole grain bread (1-1/2 slices)
rye bread (2 slices)
brown rice (1 cup cooked)
pasta (1 cup cooked)
puffed wheat (2 cups)

Note: Many of these carbohydrates also contain protein.

Quick Conversions
1/8 teaspoon . . . . a pinch
1 tablespoon . . . . 3 teaspoons
1/8 cup . . . . 2 tablespoons
1/4 cup . . . . 4 tablespoons
1/3 cup . . . . 5 1/2 tablespoons
1/2 cup . . . 8 tablespoons . . 4 ounces
1 pint . . . . 2 cups
1 quart . . . . 4 cups
1 gallon . . . . 4 quarts
1 ounce . . . . 2 tablespoons
28.3 grams . . . . 1 ounce

More Conversions
1 gram of carbohydrate . . . . 4 calories
1 gram of protein . . . . 4 calories
1 gram of alcohol . . . . 7 calories
1 gram of fat . . . . 9 calories

Stevia Plus™ to Sugar
Stevia Plus	Sugar
1 packet	2 teaspoons
1/4 teaspoon	1 teaspoon
2 tablespoons	1/2 cup

Quick Pick Food List continued

Note: Meat, fish and eggs also contain fat, but do not contain carbohydrates. Dairy, soy and grains contain carbohydrates and some fat. Most protein powders contain little, if any, carbohydrates unless they have been sweetened.

Proteins

Meat
30 grams = 120 calories
skinless chicken breast (4 oz.)
skinless turkey breast (4 oz.)
venison (4 oz.)
buffalo (4 oz.)
ostrich (4 oz.)
lean pork (4 oz.)
flank steak (3 oz.)

Fish
30 grams = 120 calories
salmon (4 oz.)
tuna (4 oz.)
cod (4 oz.)
shrimp (6 oz.)

Protein Powders
1 tablespoon = approximately 15-17 grams of protein
whey
soy
egg albumen
milk protein isolates

Eggs, Dairy
free-range eggs (1 egg white = 6 grams of protein)
Feta cheese (1/4 cup = 6 grams of protein)
part-skim Mozzarella cheese (1/4 cup = 6 grams of protein)
low-fat cottage cheese (1/2 cup = 13 grams of protein)
non-fat yogurt (1 cup = 12 grams of protein)
skim milk (1 cup = 8 grams of protein)

Soy
soy nuts (1 oz. = 12 grams of protein)
tofu (3 oz. = 6 grams of protein)
tempeh (1/2 cup = 15 grams of protein)
soybeans (1/2 cup = 14 grams of protein)
soy milk (1 cup = 7 grams of protein)

Fats

1 tbs. = 13 grams = 120 calories

Trans-fatty acids*
hydrogenated or partially hydrogenated oils
margarine
shortening

Saturated*
butter
palm kernel oil
coconut oil

Monounsaturated
canola mayonnaise
extra virgin olive oil
expeller pressed canola oil
olives
avocados
natural peanut butter
slivered almonds
almond butter
high oleic safflower oil
high oleic sunflower oil

Omega 3
flaxmeal
flaxseed oil
fish oils
walnuts

Omega 6
evening primrose oil
borage oil
pumpkin seed oil
soybean oil
sesame seed oil

* Eliminate or minimize these fats in your diet

Chapter 16

Step 6
Improve the Quality of the Food You Eat

The ripest peach is highest on the tree.
– James Whitcomb Riley

Take small steps when improving your nutritional plan. Over time, these small steps become a permanent part of your normal way of eating. If you make no other change, improving the quality of the foods you eat makes a tremendous difference in how you feel and look and in your overall health.

To improve the quality of your food, be conscious of what you buy at the grocery store. Read labels and buy foods in their most natural state.

Incremental Changes

Let's see how you can improve the quality of your food over time. I'll use myself as an example. When I was in college, my typical breakfast was

sugared cereal	white bread toast with butter and cinnamon
2% milk	orange juice

Compare that breakfast—full of refined carbohydrates and minimal protein— with today's breakfast.

oatmeal (Rolled Oats)	flaxseed oil, flaxmeal or walnuts
soy milk	raisins or strawberries
one-half scoop of soy protein powder or three free-range egg whites and one yolk	

This transition happened slowly. I experimented with foods and gradually improved the quality of the carbohydrates, proteins and fats in my diet. With each change, I enjoyed more satisfaction, greater energy and better mood throughout the day. I also enjoy this breakfast. I can't imagine reverting to my old college breakfast. If you told me 25 years ago, however, that I would be eating uncooked oatmeal, soy milk, flaxseed oil, protein powder or egg whites I would have said, "No way! Are you nuts?"

Let's look at some of the incremental steps you can take to improve the quality of your food.

Steps to Improve Breakfast		
Week 1	**Week 6**	**Week 12**
2 cups of coffee	1 cup of coffee	1 cup of coffee
cream (for coffee)	skim milk (for coffee)	skim or soy milk (for coffee)
bagel	1/2 bagel	1/2 bagel
cream cheese	natural peanut butter	natural peanut butter
	1/2 orange	1/2 orange or 1/2 cup berries
	water	2 free-range eggs
		water

Now look at some similar progressions for lunch whether eating out or packing your lunch. We'll incorporate small, steady changes and show the progress from week 1 through weeks 6 and 12.

Steps to Improve Lunch—Eating Out		
Week 1	**Week 6**	**Week 12**
hamburger	broiled chicken sandwich	chicken breast
French fries	side salad	vegetables
	fat-free vinaigrette	2 small redskin potatoes
		extra virgin olive oil on potatoes
soda pop	diet soda pop	water

Steps to Improve Lunch—Brown Bag		
Week 1	**Week 6**	**Week 12**
white bread	enriched wheat bread	whole grain bread
packaged lunchmeat	deli turkey	turkey breast or tuna
mayonnaise	fat-free mayonnaise	canola mayonnaise
candy bar	iceberg lettuce	Romaine lettuce, broccoli slaw and grape tomatoes
	applesauce	apple
soda pop	juice drink	water

In any of these examples, the timing may be faster or slower depending on your goals and your choices.

Improving the quality of your food can be challenging. With the prevalence of convenience and fast foods, it is easy to eat low-quality, low-nutrient foods. The more refined the food, the lower the quality. Be prepared to shop smarter and look for quality in the foods you choose. Make special requests when you are dining out to get exactly what you want.

Exert your influence as a consumer. Because health-conscious consumers exert influence, we now have many healthy products, such as free-range eggs, organic produce and soy milk in traditional stores. The chart below shows how to progress from lower-quality to higher-quality foods.

Poor	Better	Best
margarine	butter	non-hydrogenated butter flavored spread
olive oil	virgin olive oil	extra virgin olive oil
refined peanut butter		natural peanut butter
iceberg lettuce		Romaine lettuce, spinach
whole milk	2% milk	skim milk or soy milk
fried chicken	baked chicken thighs	baked free-range chicken breast
juice drink	fruit juice	whole fruit

Food Target

Learning to improve the quality of the foods you eat is the essence of the Meal Patterning program. Use the food target as a learning tool and a lifelong guide for eating. The food target places the lowest-quality foods on the outer rings of the target. These are the foods that are the least nourishing and can be detrimental to your health. The most beneficial, highest-quality foods—those that make the body stronger—are closer to the center of the target. You will find unrefined, natural foods closer to the center of the food target. Think about what you plan to eat. Is it a carbohydrate, protein, fat or a combination of all three? Think about the quality of the foods. Do they belong along the outer rings of the food target or toward the center? Write down your food choices in the blank food target and analyze where they fall. Compare your food target with the sample food target to evaluate your selections. By using the food target, you learn to identify carbohydrates, proteins, fats and the quality of these macronutrients.

The idea behind the Meal Patterning program is to achieve balanced eating around the target, concentrating your meals as closely as possible to the center of the target. Start slowly and make small changes.

Food Target

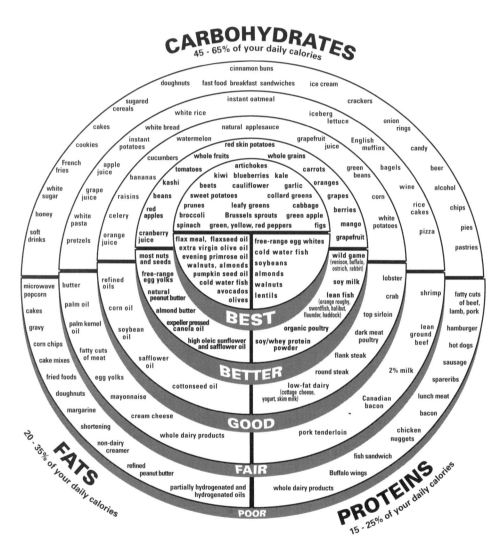

Chapter 17

Step 7

Understanding Food Combinations

What wisdom can you find that is greater than kindness?
– Jean-Jacques Rousseau

Try to balance the carbohydrates, proteins and fats every time you eat. The ideal balance is 45 to 65 percent of calories from unrefined carbohydrates, 15 to 25 percent of calories from lean proteins and 20 to 35 percent of calories from quality fats.

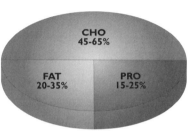

Do you have quality carbohydrates, proteins and fats? If the answer is no, add or delete foods to create better quality and balance. Start slowly and make gradual changes to each meal or snack.

Breakfast

Sample Breakfast – Poor Balance, Poor Quality			
	Carbohydrate	Protein	Fat
coffee	0 g	0 g	0 g
sugared cereal	45 g	2 g	1.5 g
whole milk	12 g	8 g	8 g
2 slices toast w/margarine	40 g	2 g	12 g
TOTALS 630 calories	**97 g** 388 calories	**12 g** 48 calories	**21.5 g** 193.5 calories
BALANCE	**61% CHO**	**8% PRO**	**31% FAT**

In the example above, there are too many calories, refined carbohydrates (sugared cereal, white bread), poor-quality fats (whole milk, butter) and little protein. Let's make it better.

Start by replacing sugared cereal with rolled oats. Switch from whole milk to soy milk (you'll be surprised how good soy milk tastes). Delete the white bread. Add raisins for increased potassium and fiber. Finally, add high-quality fat (walnuts). There are fewer calories, more vitamins, fiber and higher-quality foods.

Sample Breakfast – Improved Balance, Good Quality			
	Carbohydrate	Protein	Fat
water	0 g	0 g	0 g
rolled oats	27 g	4 g	3 g
soy milk	6 g	6 g	3 g
raisins	15 g	0 g	0 g
walnuts	2 g	2 g	7 g
TOTALS 365 calories	**50 g** 200 calories	**12 g** 48 calories	**13 g** 117 calories
BALANCE	**55% CHO**	**13% PRO**	**32% FAT**

Lunch

Sample Lunch – Good Balance, Poor Quality			
	Carbohydrate	Protein	Fat
tuna	0 g	22 g	1 g
white bread	20 g	2 g	1 g
light mayonnaise	0 g	0 g	10 g
salad	22 g	2 g	1 g
fat-free dressing	18 g	0 g	0 g
diet pop	0 g	0 g	0 g
TOTALS 461 calories	**60 g** 240 calories	**26 g** 104 calories	**13 g** 117 calories
BALANCE	**52% CHO**	**23% PRO**	**25% FAT**

In the example above, we have poor quality carbohydrates and fats and very low nutritional value. Let's make a few changes.

Sample Lunch – Good Balance, Good Quality			
	Carbohydrate	Protein	Fat
tuna	0 g	22 g	1 g
salad	22 g	2 g	1 g
sliced strawberries	20 g	0 g	0 g
balsamic vinegar & extra virgin olive oil	2 g	0 g	10 g
slivered almonds	4 g	4 g	5 g
water with lemon	0 g	0 g	0 g
TOTALS 457 calories	**48 g** 192 calories	**28 g** 112 calories	**17 g** 153 calories
BALANCE	**42% CHO**	**25% PRO**	**33% FAT**

We have improved all areas of this lunch; first, by deleting the white bread and mayonnaise, and second, by replacing the fat-free dressing with balsamic vinegar and extra virgin olive oil (good fat). We added sliced strawberries and slivered almonds for more fiber, vitamins and minerals. We replaced the diet soda pop with water and a slice of lemon. This lunch has higher-quality foods, is healthier, more satisfying and more energy-sustaining.

Dinner

We can show the same improvements for a dinner meal.

Sample Dinner – Poor Balance, Poor Quality			
	Carbohydrate	Protein	Fat
beef tips/gravy	0 g	46 g	30 g
noodles	30 g	4 g	2 g
2 rolls w/butter	35 g	4 g	20 g
corn	35 g	4 g	2 g
fat-free frozen yogurt	25 g	2 g	0 g
diet soda pop	0 g	0 g	0 g
TOTALS 1,226 calories	**125 g** 500 calories	**60 g** 240 calories	**54 g** 486 calories
BALANCE	**40% CHO**	**20% PRO**	**40% FAT**

Any time you eat this many calories (1,226) and an overabundance of refined carbohydrates (noodles, rolls and frozen yogurt) at one meal, your insulin levels will skyrocket and fat storage is inevitable. This meal has too many refined carbohydrates, too much protein and the fat content is predominantly from saturated fats. And there's just too much food. Let's see how we can clean this meal up.

Sample Dinner – Improved Balance, Good Quality			
	Carbohydrate	Protein	Fat
flank steak	0 g	30 g	6 g
2 redskin potatoes	30 g	1 g	0 g
1-1/2 cups asparagus	20 g	1 g	0 g
1 tbs extra virgin olive oil	0 g	0 g	10 g
water	0 g	0 g	0 g
TOTALS 472 calories	**50 g** 200 calories	**32 g** 128 calories	**16 g** 144 calories
BALANCE	**42% CHO**	**27% PRO**	**31% FAT**

Start off by replacing the beef tips with flank steak, which is very lean and tastes great. Then substitute redskin potatoes and asparagus for the refined carbohydrates (noodles and rolls) and replace the butter with extra virgin olive oil. Once again, notice the substitution of water for soda pop. The result: a healthy, balanced, great-tasting meal with 754 fewer calories.

Snacks

The same balance should apply to your daily snacks.

Sample Snack – Poor Balance, Poor Quality			
	Carbohydrate	Protein	Fat
pretzels	25 g	1 g	1 g
diet soda pop	0 g	0 g	0 g
TOTALS 113 calories	**25 g** 100 calories	**1 g** 4 calories	**1 g** 9 calories
BALANCE	**88% CHO**	**4% PRO**	**8% FAT**

With this snack, we once again see a high percentage of carbohydrates, low protein and low fat. It's poorly balanced and consists of poor quality foods. This snack will do little to support your energy or your health. Let's make it better.

Sample Snack – Improved Balance, Good Quality			
	Carbohydrate	Protein	Fat
smoothie drink	24 g	11 g	6 g
TOTALS 194 calories	**24 g** 96 calories	**11 g** 44 calories	**6 g** 54 calories
BALANCE	**49% CHO**	**23% PRO**	**28% FAT**

CJ's Special Smoothie

Makes three 12 oz. servings

3 cups water
2 scoops soy or whey protein powder
1 bag frozen unsweetened berries (16 oz.)

1 banana
1-1/2 tbs. flaxseed oil

Put all ingredients in blender and mix about 1 minute. Keep refrigerated.

This is a great snack for breakfast, at work, while traveling or after your work-out. With this balanced drink, you get quality carbohydrates, protein and fat for only 194 calories in a 12-ounce drink. See the recipe section for other smoothie recipes.

Consider substituting higher-quality foods at any meal or snack. Even dessert presents an opportunity to improve the balance and quality of your foods.

Stand-Alone Foods

There will be situations where you won't have an opportunity to balance your meals. If you are going to eat a carbohydrate, protein or fat by itself, try to eat it in its most natural state. A piece of fruit or a handful of nuts are great stand-alone foods. Do the best you can with what's available.

Chapter 18

Step 8
Plan Daily

There is only one corner of the universe you can be
certain of improving, and that's your own self.
— Aldous Huxley

Planning plays a critical role in successfully developing healthy nutritional patterns. Plan what you'd like to eat for breakfast, lunch, dinner and snacks. Go to the grocery store with your plan. This takes a little bit of time and effort in the beginning, but your actions soon become patterns.

Food Preparation

The key to consistently healthy eating is food preparation. I rarely leave the house without packing a few meals or snacks, especially if I am going to be gone for the entire day. The excuse I commonly hear from frustrated clients is, "I don't have time to make breakfast or prepare foods for the day." If mornings are too busy for food preparation, take ten minutes the night before and pack healthy foods for the next day. It doesn't take long to get your food ready, and you will have healthy, energy-sustaining food at your fingertips.

Developing healthy eating patterns is the essence of Meal Patterning. For those of you who think you don't have time to eat breakfast, try mixing a smoothie drink the night before. It not only tastes great, but gets your day off to a great start.

The key to easy food preparation is having the right equipment and ingredients.

- **Purchase a food steamer.** It's great for steaming vegetables, potatoes, eggs, rice and oatmeal.

- **Purchase a good blender.** Look for one with a wide bottom. A blender is great for mixing up smoothie drinks and other recipes, like oatmeal and power protein pancakes.

- **Buy a small cooler with plastic containers for travel or to take to work.**

- **Experiment with foods you like and make them easy to eat.** I enjoy a big salad at lunch, so I buy bags of prewashed spinach and broccoli slaw and throw them into a re-sealable plastic bowl. I add tuna or chicken breast, walnuts, raisins and a dressing of extra virgin olive oil and balsamic vinegar. This takes me less than five minutes to prepare. I take this to work, or toss it together at home for a fast, easy, healthy meal.

- **Take that extra ten minutes to fix daily meals—breakfast, lunch and snacks.** The ten minutes invested in planning and preparation will pay huge dividends in health, energy and lower body fat.

- **Keep quick and easy food sources in the house so you never lack healthy choices.** Good staples are cottage cheese, nuts, fruit, eggs and yogurt.

Balanced Eating While on the Run

In our fast-paced lives, it is difficult to have balance in our meals. On the right are a few ways to improve the balance of snacks while eating on the run. Don't worry about exact proportions. The idea is to incorporate foods that give a good balance of carbohydrates, protein and quality fat.

Healthy Snack	Healthy Snack w/Improved Balance
low-fat cottage cheese	add almonds, walnuts or flaxseed oil
whole-grain bread	add natural peanut or almond butter
apple slices	add natural peanut or almond butter
low-fat yogurt	add flaxseed oil and fruit
tuna in water	add canola mayonnaise, broccoli slaw & walnuts
oatmeal and raisins	add almonds or walnuts (like trail mix)
fruit smoothie drink	add flaxseed oil and protein powder

Making Smart Restaurant Menu Choices

Eating out is one of the most popular leisure activities in the United States. According to the National Restaurant Association, a trade group representing 844,000 restaurants in the U.S., the average number of restaurant meals purchased per person in the year 2000 was 141—up 25 percent from 113 in 1985. With the rapid growth of chain restaurants, especially the quick-service types, eating out is now an everyday event for many Americans.

From a health standpoint, eating out can be a bit more challenging than eating at home. It is possible, however, to eat out and maintain healthy habits. Many restaurants have healthy choices, and the choices you make have a major impact on your health and waistline.

Let's look at a few examples. Let's say you have made the commitment to Meal Patterning. You're doing great—planning your meals and snacks—and then it hits you: the dreaded fast-food restaurant. You've been busy running around, forgetting to plan or simply find yourself in one of those rare situations where you have no control. You're hungry and need to eat. What do you do? Look over the menu and think each choice through carefully. Consider how you can eat healthy and still enjoy your meal. Look for the best choices. Do they

Poor Fast-Food Choice	Better Fast-Food Choice
large hamburger	salad of lettuce or greens
French fries	chicken breast or tuna
diet pop or milkshake	olive oil or vinaigrette dressing
	water or skim milk

offer a plain salad? Can you get some type of protein, like a chicken breast, to add to the salad? Can you get oil and vinegar or a vinaigrette dressing for the salad? Think of options that will be both healthy and satisfying to you. Eating at fast food restaurants need not be a complete disaster of trans-fats and mega-calories.

In a second example, you find yourself at a restaurant and have decided to have pasta with Marinara sauce, breadsticks and a trip to the salad bar. Actually, you think you are making good choices because these seem to be fairly low-fat choices. You can make it much better. Note that this meal is very high in carbohydrates (80 percent), low in protein and low in quality fat, especially if you choose that Ranch or Thousand Island salad dressing. You may feel tired and sluggish after eating this meal. Remember, insulin is a fat/carbohydrate storing hormone and by eating too many carbohydrates at one sitting, your insulin level will rise and a drop in blood glucose will follow.

Poor Restaurant Choice	Better Restaurant Choice
pasta	pasta (take home box, split portion in half)
Marinara sauce	Marinara sauce with chicken breast on top
salad with Ranch dressing	salad with extra virgin olive oil and vinegar
breadsticks with butter	side order of steamed vegetables
diet pop	water

You can easily improve the quality and balance of this meal. First, ask for a smaller portion of pasta, or ask immediately for a take-home box and split the portion in half before eating. Second, skip the breadsticks. Breadsticks are refined carbohydrates and have little in the way of nutritional value. Ask for a side order of steamed vegetables instead. Ask to have a chicken breast or salmon filet added on top of the pasta to provide good-quality protein. Use extra virgin olive oil and vinegar on your salad and drink water.

There are many ways to create balance and improve quality when eating out. Start with a high-quality protein such as chicken, fish, soy or legumes. Choose unrefined carbohydrates such as fibrous vegetables to take the place of refined breads, crackers or pasta. Search for good fats such as extra virgin olive oil. Ask for what you want. If you don't see it on the menu, ask anyway. Most restaurants will let you make substitutions to have your meal your way.

Dining Out Tips

- Balance your carbohydrates, proteins and fats.
- Request steamed vegetables.
- Ask for a smaller portion or ask for a take-home box.
- Pass on the crackers, bread and breadsticks.
- Drink water instead of soda pop or coffee.
- Order your meat or fish grilled or broiled.

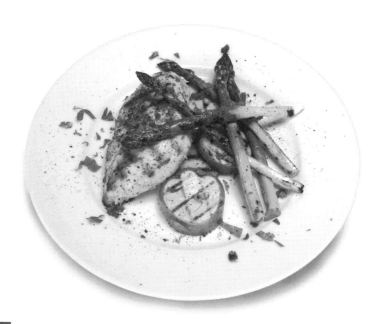

Chapter 19

Step 9
Designing Your Program

The only people who never fail are those who never try.
— Ilka Chase

When putting together your own nutritional program, experiment with different foods and recipes. I have laid out a one-week Meal Patterning plan. Each daily menu contains approximately 1,500 calories. Depending on your calorie needs (activity level, lean muscle mass, stress, frequency of meals and food quality), you may need to increase or decrease your quantity at each meal to alter your caloric intake. This is just a sample to demonstrate how to lay out your Meal Patterning program. I also give you a food log and a food target in Chapter 24. Make copies and use them as learning tools. Start slowly and make small changes.

Monday

Breakfast	**387 calories**
Oatmeal on the Run (p. 164)	
Snack	**150 calories**
1 cup yogurt with 1/2 cup fruit	
Lunch	**400 calories**
Vegetarian Roll-Up	
1 10-in. flour tortilla 1/4 cup hummus	
1/2 tomato chopped Romaine lettuce	
1/4 cup tabouli salad 1 tbs. slivered almonds (optional)	
Snack	**144 calories**
Turkey Roll-Up (p. 168)	
Dinner	**398 calories**
Grilled Salmon and Vegetables (p. 186)	
Total calories 1,479	

Tuesday

Breakfast	194 calories
CJ's Special Smoothie (p. 169)	
Snack	170 calories
1/2 to 2/3 cup low-fat cottage cheese with fruit of choice	
Lunch	276 calories
Chicken Salad (p. 172)	
Snack	200 calories
Energized Bars - 1 bar (p. 168)	
Dinner	284 calories
Mexican Pizza (p. 184)	
Snack	170 calories
Easy Egg Whites (p. 168)	

Total calories 1,294

Wednesday

Breakfast	350 calories
cereal (1/2 cup rolled oats or 2/3 cup dry cereal)	
1 tbs slivered almonds, walnuts or flaxmeal	
1/2 cup fruit of choice	
1/2 cup skim or soy milk	
Snack	150 calories
1 tbs walnuts	
1/2 cup grapes	
Lunch	400 calories
sandwich	
2 slices whole grain bread / 3 oz. turkey, chicken or tuna	
tomato, Romaine lettuce, onion / mustard or canola mayonnaise	
1/2 cup low-fat cottage cheese	
Snack	194 calories
CJ's Special Smoothie (p. 169)	
Dinner	346 calories
Salmon Salad (p. 174)	

Total calories 1,440

Thursday

Breakfast	275 calories
I slice toasted whole grain bread I tbs. natural peanut butter or almond butter 1/2 apple I hard boiled free-range egg	
Snack	**200 calories**
1/2 to I cup yogurt mixed with 1/2 cup fruit and I tbs. flaxseed oil	
Lunch	**264 calories**
Cherry Chicken Salad (p. 172)	
Snack	**200 calories**
Energized Bars - I bar (p. 168)	
Dinner	**336 calories**
Ostrich Soup (p. 177)	
Snack	**314 calories**
KJ's Chocolate Smoothie (p. 169)	

Total calories 1,589

Friday

Breakfast	292 calories
Heart Healthy Granola (p. 164)	
Snack	**194 calories**
CJ's Special Smoothie (p. 169)	
Lunch	**367 calories**
CJ's Big Salad (p. 174)	
Snack	**201 calories**
Yogurt Crunch (p. 170)	
Dinner	**435 calories**
Chicken and Vegetable Pizza (p. 183)	

Total calories 1,489

Saturday

Breakfast	250 calories
Egg White Omelet (p. 165)	
fruit of choice	
Snack	256 calories
Trail Mix (p. 171)	
Lunch	325 calories
grilled chicken breast	
Black Bean Mango Salad (p. 173)	
Snack	170 calories
Easy Egg Whites (p. 168)	
Dinner	425 calories
Salmon Patties (p. 186)	
redskin potatoes (baked or mashed)	
kale (sautéed in extra virgin olive oil and garlic)	
Dessert	192 calories
Cookies That "Rock" (p. 192) - 2 cookies	
4 oz. glass of skim or soy milk (optional)	

Total calories 1,618

Sunday

Breakfast	294 calories
Oatmeal Pancakes (p. 166)	
Snack	200 calories
1/2 cup yogurt mixed with	
1/2 cup mixed fruit	
1 tbs. flaxseed oil	
Lunch (Sat. night leftovers)	425 calories
Salmon Patties (p. 186)	
redskin potatoes (baked or mashed)	
kale (sautéed in extra virgin olive oil and garlic)	
Snack	140 calories
Turkey Roll-Up (p. 168)	
Dinner	425 calories
Chicken Stir-Fry (p. 184)	
serve over whole grain rice (2/3 cup)	

Total calories 1,484

Chapter 20

Step 10
Exercise–The Fountain of Youth

A will finds a way.

– Orison Swett Marden

How Much Exercise is Enough?

By now, almost everyone knows that regular exercise is good for you. Your doctor, friends, family, billboards, books, TV, radio and health professionals recommend regular exercise for whatever ails you. A report from the Surgeon General states that a sedentary lifestyle carries the same risk as smoking, high cholesterol, diabetes or high blood pressure. The research on the benefits of regular exercise is overwhelming. If exercise came in a pill, it would be the most prescribed drug in the world. Yet, even with all this knowledge, research and promotion, the United States remains a sedentary nation. Only 25 percent of the adult U.S. population exercises on a regular basis (two or three times per week).

Given everything we know, why aren't we exercising more? Over the last 20 years, I have given this question a lot of thought. I have talked with friends, family, clients, physicians and colleagues and have concluded that there are many reasons, and even more excuses, why Americans are not exercising. I believe that one reason is lack of knowledge about proper exercise. Just as with the nutritional side of the health equation, many people lack the knowledge about what to do, how to start and how much exercise is enough.

You might immediately want to challenge me. You might say, "Are you kidding? Everywhere I look there are articles, books, magazines, videos, infomercials—you name it—dedicated to exercise." And like nutrition, there's so much information that people are overwhelmed. Many people are confused about whether to do cardiovascular exercise to lose weight, high- or low-intensity to lose fat, specific exercises to shape or sculpt a certain body part, whether strength training is really necessary and how much time should be devoted to what types of exercises. In addition to these concerns, many people have specific questions about exercise that relate to their personal needs, such as, "If I have bad knees or a bad back, what can I do and what exercises should I avoid?"

I see evidence of the lack of knowledge and an abundance of misinformation everywhere. When visiting other health clubs throughout the country, working out in hotels, listening to friends, fielding questions from participants in my seminars and working in my own health club, I hear comments and rationales that people have constructed from myriad sources.

I even see it in my own family. While visiting my sister in Chicago years ago, she complained of pain in her shoulders. As we talked, she explained that her current exercise program consisted of following an exercise video two or three times a week, for 30–45 minutes, that included a combination of cardiovascular and strength training exercises.

After watching her exercise video, I explained to her that her shoulder pain was due to overuse and poor posture. Her exercise video worked the front of her shoulder (anterior deltoid) but didn't work the opposing muscle groups. We made a few small changes to her program. We deleted her standing chest fly, upright rows and shoulder press, and added a tubing wide pull (see page 133) and improved her posture. Her shoulder pain disappeared within a few weeks. I see so many people invest their precious time on exercise routines that provide them little benefit, and often put them at risk for injury.

The Bionic Woman

Let me tell you about my mother, who I call the "bionic woman." At 69 years of age, she had suffered through an ankle fusion and replacements of both hips and a knee, all within the prior five years. She had never been an exerciser, although she was fairly active as a young adult. After going through post-surgical physical therapy, I nagged her about starting a regular exercise program. She resisted, arguing that she was in too much pain and didn't have the energy to devote to exercise. She also believed that exercise would be too painful and she didn't have confidence that it would help her.

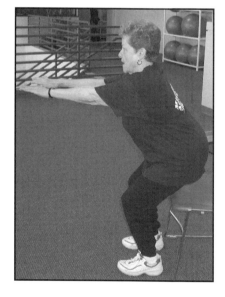

I finally convinced her to work with Todd Yehl, Co-director of Personal Training, at my home club. I'm lucky to work with Todd, who I believe is one of the best personal trainers in the United States. After working with Todd twice a week for six weeks, my mother felt noticeably less pain and had more energy. More importantly, for the first time in many years, she had hope that her physical condition could improve. Along with improved mobility, and living life with less pain, perhaps the greatest reward has been the change in my mom's attitude. She is more active, smiles all the time, talks all the time and has had her vitality restored. In addition, she is a true believer in taking her flaxseed oil (1-1/2 tablespoons a day). She extols the benefits of flaxseed oil to anyone who will listen.

I don't want to suggest that there is only one specific way to exercise, or that the exercises I discuss in this book are the only means to achieving the results you are seeking. There are endless ways to move the body and that's all that exercise is—moving your body. Yoga, cardiovascular exercise machines such as treadmills or stair climbers, swimming, walking, biking, pilates, tai chi, strength training with free weights, rubber tubing or weight-training machines are just a sampling of the exercises you can do on your own. Then there are the group activities like tennis, basketball, soccer, playing with your kids and exercise classes of many varieties. For most of us, doing the same type of exercise day in and day out can get quite boring, both mentally and physically, making it less likely we will include regular exercise in our lives.

In addition, when you do the same exercises with the same intensity, your body begins to adapt to this exercise program, or routine, very quickly. Over time, you will not see as many improvements as you did in the beginning unless you change your exercise program by finding new ways to exercise or changing the intensity of the program. The point is, change is good. Variety is healthy, both mentally and physically.

A few years ago, while skiing in Aspen, Colorado, I rode up the chair lift with a man and we began talking. He asked me what I did for a living and I explained that I worked in the health and fitness industry, educating people about eating and exercise. He told me that his wife "liked that kind of stuff" and was a member of the athletic club in Aspen. When I asked him about his exercise habits, he told me that he skis about one hundred days a year and works as a fishing guide in the Maroon Bells during the summer. As I watched him ski away, smoothly and gracefully, it hit me that his whole approach to life—his lifestyle—was tremendously active and didn't require a formal exercise program. He obviously loved what he was doing, which is very important for long-term success. By the way, this man was 72 years young.

This exercise chapter is not meant to be the be-all and end-all to your exercise program. It is meant as a starting point for the new exerciser or as a way to get back to basics for the experienced exerciser who can then incorporate greater knowledge into his or her current exercise program. **It shouldn't surprise you that I recommend hiring a personal trainer to anyone interested in starting an exercise program.** There are many wonderful personal trainers who can help you design an exercise program that fits your specific needs. Start slowly, start smart, and invest in yourself. You are worth it.

Back to Basics

When it comes to exercise, training specificity rules. If your goal is to become a marathon runner, a good portion of your exercise program must be specifically dedicated to distance running. The more specific your exercise program goals become, the greater adaptation will occur with that exercise or movement pattern. One major goal is to design a balanced program that you can enjoy. I don't say you have to love it, but it's important that you at least enjoy it!

If you are walking on the treadmill forty-five minutes a day, five days a week, with no strength training, poor posture and no stretching, you will likely develop muscle imbalances—strong muscles in the hip flexor, quadriceps and calf, with weakness in the glutes, hamstrings and upper body. One of the first goals of any exercise program is to avoid muscle imbalances in order to decrease the risk of injury and increase the ability to move better in all directions—sitting, squatting, climbing, bending, twisting and lifting.

Exercise and Weight Loss

Before I explore the specific exercise portion of this chapter, I must discuss weight loss and the mindset associated with successful weight loss. Many people I encounter have a specific goal of losing weight. Many of these folks believe that they will lose weight if they exercise more. Truth is—it just isn't that simple. You will burn more calories and maybe lose a few pounds by exercising more, but many people who exercise regularly are still overweight due to their poor nutritional patterns. Many folks also believe that long-duration, low-intensity, cardiovascular exercise is the best method to lose weight. Cardiovascular exercise is an important component of a balanced exercise program, but long-duration, low-intensity cardiovascular exercise is not the most efficient method to lose weight. The proper approach to exercise takes into account the hormonal effects that occur with exercise and includes a balanced program with moderate amounts of cardio, strength training and stretching.

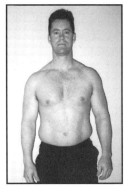
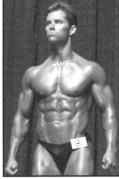

For the past few years I have competed in Natural Bodybuilding shows in the Masters Division (over age 40). My exercise routine does not change a great deal prior to my contest. But nutritionally, everything tightens up. I eat more frequently, have smaller portion sizes and take no liberties for 10-12 weeks.

Before competition   During competition

The point of showing these two photos is that my exercise routine stays virtually the same.

Proper nutritional patterns account for 80 to 85 percent of successful weight loss. To get the weight loss results you desire, you must begin with nutritional changes. Interestingly, while 80 to 85 percent of initial weight loss begins with nutrition, research shows that 75 percent of *maintaining* weight loss has to do with other lifestyle factors, the most important being regular exercise. Regular exercise is critical for long-term weight control combined with maintenance of proper nutritional patterns.

Posture Alignment

When I was young, my grandmother always told me to "stand up straight and tall." She was right to stress the benefits of good posture. What is ideal posture alignment and why is it so important? Ideal posture alignment happens when the body is perfectly aligned, or in neutral position, starting with the feet and ankles, and moving up through the knees, hips, pelvis, arms, shoulders, neck and head.

As we age, we are in a constant battle with gravity, which is working to pull us out of ideal, or neutral, posture alignment. Daily stresses of life, sitting, standing, bending, walking, playing and exercising challenge our ideal posture alignment. We all make some type of compromise when it comes to our posture. The challenge, and the goal, is to identify our own ways of compromising and correct them, trying to improve our posture alignment.

This is where exercise can be especially beneficial. We all get into repetitive movement patterns and, over time, certain muscles become shorter and stronger, while opposing muscles may become longer and weaker, creating muscle imbalance that leads to poor posture, injury, pain and decreased mobility. Proper exercise improves muscle imbalances and leads to better posture alignment.

Many older males who come to me for training complain of back pain, knee pain, tight hips and weakness in their legs. Many have what I call the "TV repairman syndrome," or disappearing glutes. Every time they sit or bend over, they hinge at the knees or lower back, without using the muscles in their hips and glutes. The load is placed in the lower back and knees, causing pain in both areas. The solution: retrain the mind to fire the muscles of the glutes and hips. Learn the perfect technique by doing a chair squat or a stride lunge, or both. This will improve posture, get the muscles to work in the correct sequence, thus decreasing pain in the knees and lower back.

I see many women who have pain, weakness and discomfort in their shoulders, upper back and neck, and many complain of frequent headaches. I immediately explain to them they are waging a battle with gravity and try to inspire them to fight back. Gravity wins this battle when the shoulders begin to round and the head is moved forward, causing unusual stress on the muscles supporting the head, neck, shoulders and upper back. Strengthening the muscles of the middle back, elevating the rib cage and pulling the shoulders back and down will create a more ideal posture alignment. In turn, this will reduce the stress on the muscles of the neck, shoulders and upper back, ultimately decreasing the pain and frequency of headaches.

Every exercise should begin with ideal posture alignment. The challenge is to maintain ideal posture during the exercise. The discipline of thinking about ideal posture in a formal exercise program helps focus our thinking on proper posture alignment during everyday life—walking, sitting, driving, working and sleeping. Everywhere you go, during all of your day's activities, try to maintain the best posture you can and remember the admonition of my grandmother to "stand up straight and tall."

Components of a
Balanced Exercise Program

As I mentioned earlier, there are many ways to exercise, but keep in mind the importance of finding exercise that is both enjoyable and balanced.

There are four basic components of a balanced exercise program.

1. Warm-up (dynamic stretching)

2. Cardiovascular exercise

3. Strength training

4. Stretching and flexibility

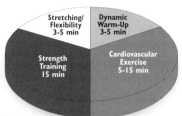

Although each of the four components will be discussed separately, they can cross over and be integrated as one. For example, power yoga combines all four components in one workout. But remember, training specificity rules. If your goal is to become a competitive body builder or an elite endurance athlete, you will not achieve it doing power yoga. If integrated into an athlete's exercise program, however, power yoga can enhance it overall, create better balance and decrease the chance of injuries.

Warm-up

With every form of exercise, you need a time to transition from a static or sedentary state into a dynamic or active state, activating the nervous, cardiovascular and muscular systems. I use dynamic stretching exercises (see pages 124-126) before I play tennis, ski, golf or do strength training or any other form of exercise. Dynamic stretches cover the entire body, improve balance and flexibility and are quick (take three to five minutes to complete). Use slow and controlled movements and gradually increase the range of motion as you warm up. If there are movements that are difficult, let pain be your guide and modify those movements. Do not continue a warm-up exercise that is causing you pain. Start with the smaller muscle groups and gradually begin to work the large muscles.

Cardiovascular Exercise

When most people think of cardiovascular exercise, they think of walking, jogging, biking, swimming, cross-country skiing, inline skating—virtually any exercise that is rhythmic in nature. It is true that these are all forms of cardiovascular exercise. Cardiovascular exercise places demands on the heart, lungs and muscles. There are many benefits including stress reduction, reduced insulin levels, mood elevation, increased cardiovascular efficiency, decreased blood pressure, improved blood lipids and weight control.

Cardiovascular exercise can be either aerobic or anaerobic depending on the intensity level of the exercise.

> Aerobic exercise = supply of oxygen meets demand of the exercise
>
> Anaerobic exercise = demand of the exercise exceeds the supply of oxygen

It is important to understand the difference between aerobic and anaerobic exercises and how the intensity of your exercise program can affect certain hormones and, more importantly, help you get the results you desire. Your "fountain of youth" hormones, testosterone (produced by both men and women) and growth hormone, are stimulated by higher intensity anaerobic exercise. These two hormones help the body get leaner, stronger and more youthful.

When educating my clients about cardiovascular exercise, I explain that as their cardiovascular fitness levels start to improve, the goal is not to increase the length of time dedicated to cardiovascular exercise, but to slowly increase the intensity level, or difficulty, of that exercise.

Many people look at cardiovascular exercise as a way to burn calories and decrease body fat, assuming that more is better. This is not necessarily true. If your goal is weight loss, it is far more effective and more efficient to limit the time spent on cardiovascular exercise to 15-20 minutes, but raise the intensity. The higher intensity, and corresponding stimulation of testosterone and growth hormone, will have a far greater impact on weight loss than tracking the number of calories burned.

It sounds simple. To lose weight using cardiovascular exercise, increase the intensity and go like mad! But hold on. There are a few things you must understand about high-intensity cardiovascular exercise. First, if your intensity level becomes too high, your lean hormones begin to disappear and the stress hormone cortisol comes out in their place. Cortisol is the major stress hormone that beats the body up and breaks it down. The effects of cortisol are opposite those of testosterone and growth hormone. Cortisol ages the body faster than any other hormone. It decreases bone density and increases the risk of heart disease, cancer, muscle wasting and fat storage.

Second, it is more difficult to keep ideal posture alignment with higher intensity cardiovascular exercise. Poor postural alignment may lead to orthopedic problems and injuries.

If you enjoy going for a leisurely long walk or bike ride (30-60 minutes), do it and enjoy all the wonderful benefits that follow. But if your goal is weight loss, start adding some short bouts of higher-intensity effort throughout your cardiovascular exercise program as you become more efficient with your exercise time. The benefits of cardiovascular exercise do not increase by adding more time to your program. 15-20 minutes of moderate- to high-intensity cardiovascular exercise are all that's needed. Adding more time can lead to orthopedic problems and stimulate the wrong hormones (cortisol and adrenaline).

Clients tell me that one of the main barriers to regular exercise is lack of time. Time is precious. Don't waste it with unnecessary cardiovascular exercise. Unless your goal is to participate in endurance activities such as long distance marathon running or triathlons, stick with short duration, higher-intensity cardiovascular exercise. Start slowly and progress gradually to allow your body adequate time to adapt to the demands of exercise.

Cardiovascular exercise outline

1. **Modality:** It's what you do. Find an exercise you enjoy and add variety to your workouts. Walking, biking, swimming, running, hiking, snowshoeing, cross-country skiing and using cardiovascular machines are just a few of the good cardiovascular exercises that many people enjoy.

2. **Frequency:** It's how often you do it. Try to develop exercise patterns that fit your available time and schedule. Exercise two to five times a week. Start slowly.

3. **Duration:** It's how long you do it. Just 10 minutes of cardiovascular exercise has benefits. Ideally, try to get in 15-20 minutes and pay attention to posture and intensity level. Focus on your goals and be efficient with your time.

4. **Intensity:** It's how hard you work. "Intensity" means the level of difficulty in sustaining the exercise. If the exercise is so hard that you can last only a few minutes before you have to quit, your intensity level is too high. If your intensity level is too low, your body will make only minimal adaptations and you will get fewer benefits from the exercise session.

Four methods to monitor exercise intensity

1. **Visually:** Watch body language and postural alignment. If intensity is too high, the body begins to make compensations leading to a breakdown in postural alignment.

2. **Talk test:** As exercise intensity increases, it becomes more difficult to talk. The body is switching energy systems from aerobic into anaerobic metabolism. If you can easily carry on a conversation your intensity may be too low. If you can only say a few words without stopping to catch your breath, your intensity is too high. Find the balance that is specific to your goals.

3. **Perceived exertion:** Assess your level of exertion on a 1-10 scale, with 1-2 being very easy, 4-6 being moderate and 8-10 being high.

4. **Heart rate:** Traditionally, this is the gold standard for monitoring exercise intensity. As exercise intensity increases, heart rate increases. Use the following formula to find a target heart rate zone. Take 220 minus your age and multiply this number by how hard you want to exercise. A beginning level, or lower-intensity level, would be 50-60 percent. The maximum or highest-intensity level is 80-90 percent. Let's figure out a heart rate zone to fit a 40-year-old person's fitness level.

Intensity	Age	Intensity	Heart Rate
Easy:	220 - 40 (age)=	180 x 50% =	90 bpm (beats per minute)
Moderate:	220 - 40 (age) =	180 x 60-70% =	108-126 bpm
High:	220 - 40 (age) =	180 x 80-90% =	144-162 bpm

If you are just getting started with exercise, start slowly and keep your heart rate around 90-100 beats per minute (bpm). For a moderate exerciser, 108-126 bpm would be the goal. For the advanced exerciser or for doing interval training, 144-162 bpm is the target. These are just guidelines. Monitor your heart rate further with the talk test and by assessing your perceived exertion to see how your heart rate measures up.

The challenge of monitoring your heart rate is that it uses age as a predictor of fitness level, which is often inaccurate. If you are on any medications, especially cardiac medications, the medication may affect heart rate levels. It's important to use all of the methods to monitor the intensity level of your exercise.

Remember to start slowly and let your body slowly acclimate to your exercise program.

Strength Training — The Fountain of Youth

If there is one form of exercise that can turn back the hands of time, it is strength training. More and more, people reap its benefits. Even people in their 80s and 90s improve their strength and bone density with strength training. I have seen firsthand the benefits of strength training with many clients who have trained with me for over ten years. Strength training is exercise that uses resistance to place demands on the nervous system, hormones, bones and muscles. Strength training is generally done with a short burst (10-30 seconds) of the strength training phase, followed by a recovery phase. The rest or recovery phase can last 10 seconds to three minutes. The benefits of strength training are increased strength, increased bone density, fewer injuries, increased self-esteem, enhanced mobility and functionality, improved posture, increased metabolism and weight loss.

With the right intensity, strength training taxes the anaerobic system and thus stimulates testosterone and growth hormone. Women, don't be afraid that you will bulk up by doing strength training. Men have more testosterone than women. It takes a tremendous amount of effort, good nutrition and the right parents for women to get larger muscles. As I tell my clients, I have been trying to get bigger muscles for 30 years and it's very difficult.

Strength training can take many forms. Your own body weight, free-weights, rubber tubing and strength-training machines are just a few. As you begin your strength-training program, focus on the following four guidelines.

1. **Ideal posture:** Before the start of each exercise, get into your ideal posture and maintain this postural alignment throughout the entire exercise. When postural alignment begins to break down, stop the exercise.

2. **Visualization:** Concentrate on the exercise you are performing and feel the muscles you are trying to work. Ask yourself if you are making a connection between the brain and the muscles, using your body's neuromuscular system. This is one of your major goals — to learn how to feel the muscles that you are targeting.

3. **Exhale during the exertional phase of each exercise:** Do not hold your breath. When doing a push-up, for example, exhale as you push your body up and inhale as you go down.

4. **Proper Progressions:** There's more to strength training than repetitions, sets and resistance. As your body adapts to your strength training program, start making a few small changes in your program so your body stays challenged and continues to make adaptations. The seven areas of proper progressions—number of exercises, sets, repetitions, resistance, rest and recovery, speed of movement, stability and balance— are described on the next page.

Number of exercises: The big question is how many exercises to do. If you are just beginning, work the entire body by doing four to six exercises. As you advance, add a few more exercises or divide your routine into splits (upper body on the first day, lower body on the second day).

Sets: Start with one set of each exercise. As you advance, move to two to four sets per exercise.

Repetitions: Within each set, do from six to 12 repetitions, or "reps." Use reps as a guideline to measure your intensity and progress. Most of my clients work in a range of eight to 12 reps per set. Choose fewer (six to 10) reps if your goal is greater resistance or load; more (12 to 15) reps if your goal is less resistance. More important than the number of reps is your technique and maintaining proper posture throughout each exercise movement. If your posture breaks down, regardless of your desired rep range, stop the exercise. Losing proper posture is how people get injured, develop muscle imbalances and poor movement patterns.

Resistance: Resistance is the load used in any given set or rep. Choosing the correct resistance can be a bit challenging at first. Your goal with every exercise is to create perfect exercise technique and then to add resistance to challenge the muscular system to maintain ideal posture and stress the working muscles. I tell my clients, "Listen to your body, maintain perfect form and don't get caught up in just pushing weight."

Rest and recovery: The more intensity, reps and resistance in each exercise set, the more recovery time will be necessary between sets. If your goal is to max out during a certain amount of resistance, you will need a longer recovery time between sets (two to three minutes). If your goal is to integrate many exercises with a moderate amount of resistance, you should have shorter recovery times (30 seconds) between sets.

Speed of movement: Speed of movement is an important tool to help monitor the intensity of each exercise. Begin with a two-second count in both phases of the strength movement, making the total time for each rep four seconds.

Stability and balance: As you improve and become more fit, start challenging your stability and balance. When you are beginning, it is much easier to strength train while you are stable, (e.g., sitting at a chest press machine as opposed to doing a push-up while your feet are up on a step or Swissball).

Follow these guidelines and focus on your ideal posture alignment. Watch as you progress and the benefits of strength training will unfold before your eyes.

Equipment Needs

Very little equipment is needed for many of the strength training exercises I recommend. Start by using your own body weight and exercise tubing. Exercise tubing comes in four colors, representing different levels of resistance. Yellow is easiest, green and red become relatively harder and blue provides the greatest level of resistance. **Gym on the Go™** is a great product, made up of all levels of tubing and an easy to follow guide. For information about Gym on the Go, visit www.gymonthego.com.

It is also a good idea to purchase a few dumbbells. A good starter set includes 5, 8, 10, 12, 15 and 20 pound dumbbells. Ultimately, the dumbbells you use will depend on your fitness level and your goals.

I also recommend purchasing a Swissball. These come in different sizes, 55 cm for people 5'8" tall or under and 65 cm for those 5'9" or taller. These balls can be purchased at your local sporting goods or fitness equipment store and are both inexpensive (typically under $25) and very versatile.

Finally, I recommend purchasing an adjustable bench and a yoga mat for floor and stretching exercises. All of your fitness equipment needs can be purchased at most exercise or fitness stores.

Stretching/Flexibility Exercises

The benefits of stretching the muscles of the body are many, from decreasing stress to improving muscle imbalances. Stretching exercises should be performed after the body is warmed up or at the end of your exercise program. There are hundreds of different stretching exercises from which to choose. I have chosen a few basic stretches that cover the entire body. Don't neglect the stretching portion of your exercise program. Start with just two or three stretching exercises and gradually build from there. Focus on proper body alignment and breathing (deep, slow breathing). Stretching exercises may be done daily. A few general rules apply to stretching.

1. **Hold each stretch for 10-60 seconds.**

2. **Maintain ideal posture throughout all stretches.**

3. **Do not stretch to a point of discomfort.**

**See Section III (Tools for Success)
for more specific exercise information.**

Chapter 21

Step 11
You Can Do It!

Change starts when someone sees the next step.
— William Drayton

Here's the real challenge: making healthy lifestyle changes a reality. Change is a process and true success comes in small increments. For some people, the concept of Meal Patterning might be initially overwhelming. It seems difficult to implement into their lives and there is a lot of information to absorb at one time. This is why it is important to break it down into steps that you can easily handle. The first step is to decide if you are ready to change any of your lifestyle habits. You might read this book and find a few small things you are ready and willing to change or, perhaps, you have already made some changes and are ready to tackle the next level. Either way, you will experience success because you will have taken a step towards a healthier way of life.

Once you have determined your level of commitment, start making Meal Patterning your own. Take a part of the program that you feel you can handle and begin to make changes. For example, study the food target and see where your current foods fall. Instead of trying to head straight for the center, gradually move one rung closer. After you have made a few small changes and are ready for more, go back and read another chapter and begin to make a few more adjustments. The people whose testimonials you've read in this book did not make their changes overnight. They moved along the continuum, gathering information and making small adjustments until they reached their goals. I have listed a few strategies that will help you make Meal Patterning your own. Take that first step and never look back!

Determine How Ready You Are for Change

Take some time now to sit down and decide what you want to change, and why. Look at where you are now and what you can realistically change. How can you make some of the suggestions in this book a reality right now? Which changes might have to wait? Do you need more information or are you ready? What part of Meal Patterning do you want to tackle first, and why? Remember, you are the driver. You choose the changes you wish to make.

- **Make Meal Patterning your own.** Make small changes that are right for you!

- **Focus on what you want to achieve.** Be specific. Create positive energy by focusing on what you **want**, not on what you don't want.

- **Use positive self-talk.** We are constantly engaging in conversation with ourselves. Whether this conversation is positive or negative has a great impact on our daily activities. Learning to look at your choices in a positive way will greatly affect your success.

- **Build on success.** By making small changes, you develop the confidence that you can do it. Keep taking small steps forward and watch your success grow.

- **Expect bumps in the road.** We all have times in our lives when we get off track. Don't let one meal, day, week or even a month of poor eating and exercise habits get you down. Don't give up. Get your focus back. Everyone has lapses now and then. Look at your successes and how you have made improvements along the ladder of health. Even if you have a lapse occasionally, very rarely will you go all the way back to where you started. Monitor yourself weekly. Are you getting enough rest? Are you moving your body regularly? Are you making good nutritional decisions? If you've slipped a little, recognize the early warning signs and get back on track toward better health.

- **Eliminate roadblocks.** Successful lifestyle change requires time, energy and other resources. If it is difficult to find time to exercise, try scheduling a regular appointment. Or, if going out to lunch every day makes staying on your plan challenging at times, try packing your lunch three days a week. Identify resources you need and eliminate barriers that get in the way of your success.

- **Stay pumped.** Staying motivated over time can be challenging for almost everyone. Find ways to keep yourself motivated to maintain healthy lifestyle habits. This is where the goals you set will encourage you. Keep your goals in sight and repeat them to yourself each day. Why are you attempting this change? If it is important, it should be motivating. Try to keep your motivators positive. Behavior change is difficult if negative feelings of guilt or shame are involved. Make a list of the benefits of exercise and eating well. Use this list each day as your motivator to stay on track. Tell yourself you are exercising today to strengthen your heart or your bones, or maybe to reduce stress or boost your immune system. If your goal is to lose weight and it does not seem to be happening as fast as you'd like, don't let it overshadow all the positive changes you are making. With positive changes come positive results.

- **Enjoy the journey.** As with any challenge, the journey is as rewarding as the outcome. You may be surprised at what you can accomplish. Enjoy the journey—you are worth it!

The Carpenter and the Contractor

An elderly carpenter was ready to retire. He told his employer-contractor of his plans to leave the house-building business and to live a more leisurely life with his family. He would miss the paycheck, but he needed to retire. The contractor was sorry to see his good worker go and asked if the carpenter could build just one more house for him as a personal favor. The carpenter said yes, but in time it was easy to see that his heart was not in his work. He resorted to shoddy workmanship and used inferior materials. It was an unfortunate way to end his career. When the carpenter finished his work and the contractor came to inspect the house, the contractor handed the front-door key to the carpenter. "This is your house," he said, "my gift to you." What a shock! What a shame! If he had only known he was building his own house, he would have done it all so differently. Now he had to live in the home he had built none too well.

So it is with us. We build our lives in a distracted way, reacting rather than acting, willing to put up with less than the best. At important points, we do not give the job our best effort. Then, with a shock we look at the situation we have created and find that we are now living in the house we have built. If we realized that, we would have done it differently.

Think of yourself as the carpenter. Think about your house. Each day you hammer a nail, place a board or erect a wall, build wisely. It is the only life you will ever build. Even if you live it only for one day more, that day says, "Life is a do-it-yourself project." Your life today is the result of your attitudes and choices in the past. Your life tomorrow will be the result of your attitude and the choices you make today.

— Author Unknown

Tools for Success
A Guide to Everyday Life

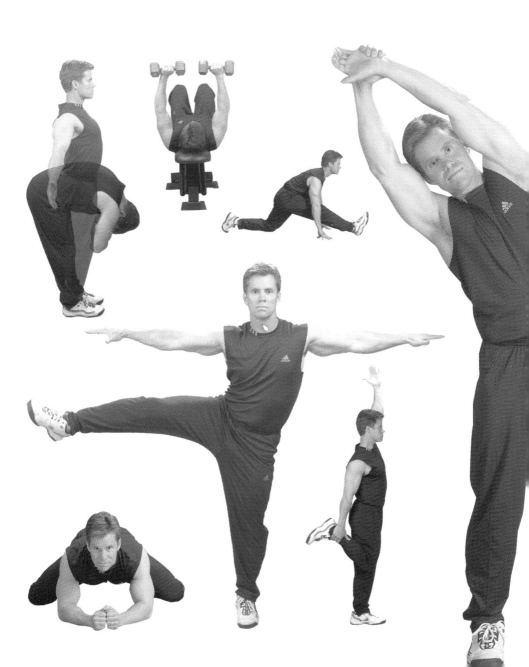

Chapter 22

Exercises–
The Fountain of Youth

Don't wait for your ship to come in, swim out to it.
– Anonymous

This section introduces you to a variety of exercises that can be completed with a minimal investment of time, equipment or expense. Use the written information on exercise in Chapter 20 along with the photos in this section. I have given you a few sample exercise routines in the back of this chapter as a start. Try to maintain a balance in your exercise program and pay attention to proper form for all exercises. Start slowly and enjoy all the benefits that regular exercise brings.

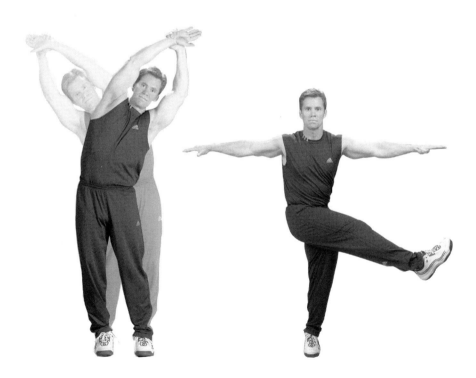

Index of Exercises

Posture

Here are a few tips to improve your posture. With every exercise you perform, your first thought should be, "Am I in ideal posture?"

- Place **feet** hip-width apart, toes pointed straight ahead. Feet should be even with each other and your weight evenly distributed.
- **Knees** should be straight but not locked (soft knees).
- **Hips** should be level with a neutral pelvis. To find neutral pelvis, rotate hips forward (tuck your tail in), rotate back (stick your glutes out) and end in the middle of these two movements. Abdominal and glute muscles should be engaged for stabilization.
- Lift your **rib cage** (chest) up, pull navel up and in, pull your shoulders back and down.
- Keep your **arms** at your sides with palms facing the body, thumbs pointing straight ahead.
- Center **head** and **neck** over your shoulders. Keep your eyes straight ahead with chin parallel to the ground.

Practice this posture daily and see what a difference ideal posture can make.

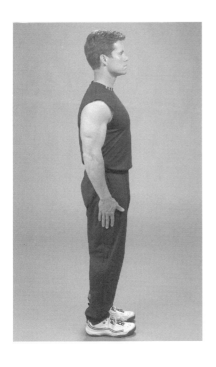
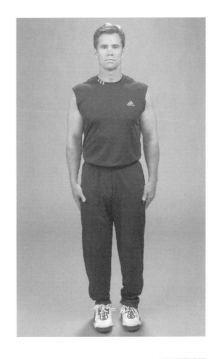

Warm-up

As with any exercise program, you need to make a slow transition from being sedentary to being active. The major goal of the warm-up phase is to increase body temperature allowing greater blood circulation, increasing the temperature of the muscles and connective tissues and increasing elasticity in the muscles (easier to move and stretch). Your warm-up should last 5–10 minutes. Fast walking or riding a stationary bike are excellent warm-up exercises.

Dynamic Stretching

Dynamic stretching is done by actively moving the body in a controlled fashion through the desired range of motion. The major advantage of dynamic stretching over static stretching before you exercise is that it engages the nervous system to activate your muscles, getting them ready to move. Start with the fingers and wrists and gradually move down the body. Do each exercise slowly and with control, for 4-10 repetitions per exercise. Dynamic stretching should take 3-5 minutes.

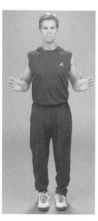 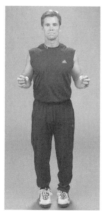 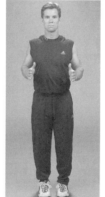

Fingers and Wrist

Bend, spread and rotate fingers. Move thumbs up and down. Move wrist up and down. Rotate wrists.

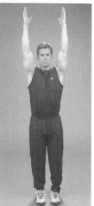 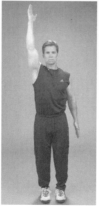 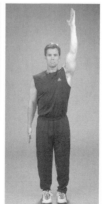

Shoulders

Alternate raising arms, palms facing each other.

Trunk

Round the Spine

As you round your spine, pull navel into your spine.

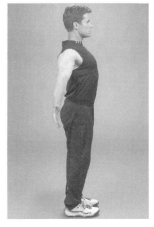
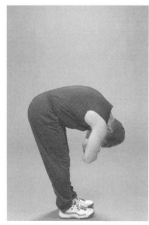

Side Bend

As you reach over, let opposite heel come up. Alternate sides.

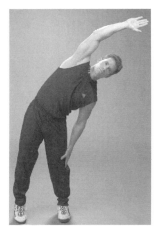
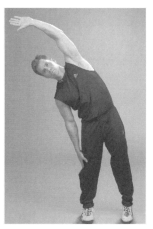

Trunk Twist

As you twist, lift heel. Twist slowly side to side.

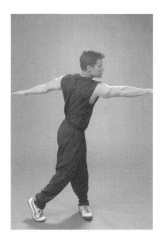
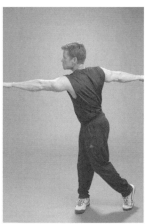

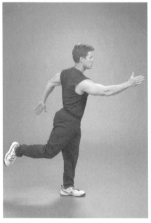
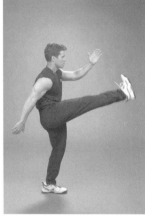

Leg Swings

Front Leg Swing

Hold on to the wall or a chair when first performing this exercise. Maintain ideal posture. With leg slightly bent, swing leg forward and back. To improve balance try this exercise without holding on.

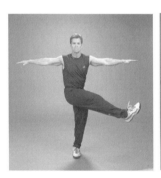
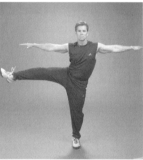

Side Leg Swing

Hold on to the wall or a chair when first performing this exercise. Maintain ideal posture. Slightly bend the knee of the support leg. Swing the opposite leg in both directions with toes pointed up. Alternate legs. To improve balance and coordination, try this exercise without holding on.

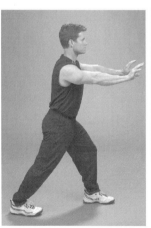
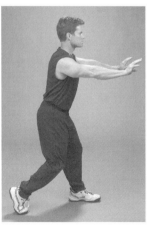

Calf Stretch

Place hands against wall. Lean into the wall. Slowly rock forward onto toes and then down, alternating legs.

Strength Training Lower Body

Chair Squat

Target Muscles:
glutes, quadriceps, hamstrings

Start in ideal posture, hands extended in front, navel up and in, and weight spread evenly between feet. Push the hips back and bend forward slowly as you squat. Pause the bend at 90 degrees. Keep knees aligned with second toe. As you slowly stand up, squeeze your glutes. To modify the movement (make it easier), decrease range of motion or hold on to counter or table.

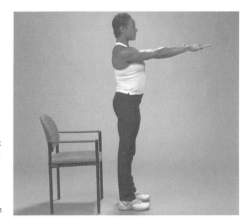

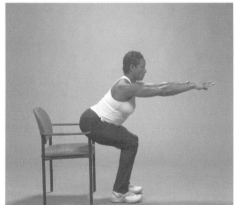

Dumbbell Squat

Target Muscles:
glutes, quadriceps, hamstrings

Perform chair squat with arms at side holding dumbbells. Keep shoulders back and navel pulled up and in.

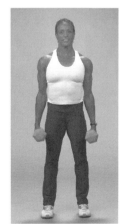

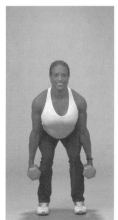

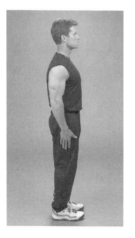
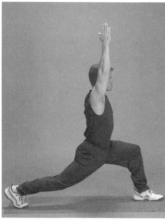

Straight Leg "Yoga" Lunge

Target Muscles: *quadriceps, glutes, hamstrings*

Start with feet shoulder-width apart. Lift the arms up while bending the knee to a 90-degree angle and slowly reaching back with the opposite leg to a wide stance lunge. Back leg is straight, glute is contracted (tight). Front leg knee is tracking over the second toe. Pull navel up and in. Don't forget to breathe. Hold this movement for 10–30 seconds. Alternate legs.

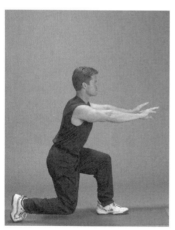
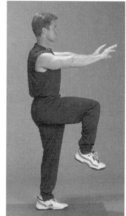

Stride Lunge

Target Muscles: *glutes, quadriceps, hamstrings*

Stand with feet shoulder-width apart, arms forward and fingertips against a mirror or wall. Reach back with right leg, keeping weight in heel of left foot and hips squared. Lower yourself slowly until left leg is bent 90 degrees and right knee is 2–3 inches off floor. Keep arms straight, chest up, shoulders down and in (imagine pinching a pencil between your shoulder blades). Hold position 2–5 seconds.

Return to standing position and raise right leg until thigh is parallel to floor and leg is bent 90 degrees, toes pointed down. Hold 2–5 seconds. Return to standing position. Alternate legs. To modify this exercise, make your movement smaller.

Tubing Side Step

Target Muscles:
glutes, hips

With glutes slightly back, navel up and in, keeping your toes square, step slowly side to side and back, keeping tension in the tubing. Keep hands on hips, chest up and shoulders back. Keep the upper body quiet (imagine balancing a cup of water on each shoulder). Remember to keep toes facing straight (forward).

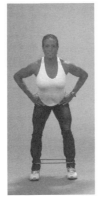 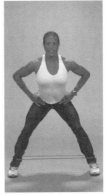 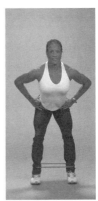

Standing Calf Raise

Target Muscles:
calves

In ideal posture position, with knees slightly bent, raise up on the toes. Hold for 2–3 seconds at the top position. To increase intensity, try not holding on to the chair. You can also do this exercise on the edge of a stair step. Hold on to the railing for support and lower the heels slightly below the level of the step.

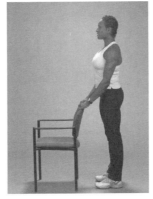 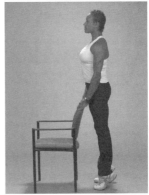

Single Leg Calf Raise

Target Muscles:
calves

Bring knee of one leg up to chest and hold. Raise up on the opposite leg, maintaining ideal posture. Alternate legs.

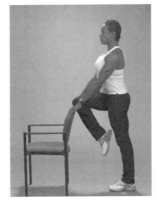 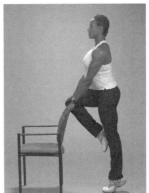

Strength Training Upper Body

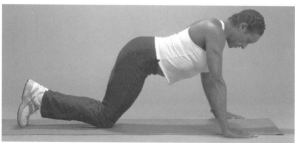

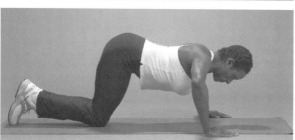

Beginner Push-up

Target Muscles:
chest, triceps, anterior deltoid

Start with knees together, toes touching the floor, hips up, navel pulled up and in, and hands slightly wider than shoulder width. Keeping shoulder blades together and hips up and over knees, slowly lower chest until elbows form a 90-degree angle while inhaling. Keeping elbows out, hold, then push from chest to bring body back to start position. Exhale as you push up.

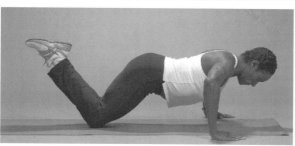

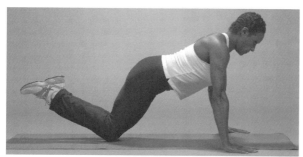

Modified Push-up

Target Muscles:
chest, triceps, anterior deltoid

Start with knees together, toes off the floor, hips up, navel pulled up and in, and hands slightly wider than shoulder width. Keeping shoulder blades together, lower chest until elbows form a 90-degree angle while inhaling. Keeping elbows out, hold, then push from chest to bring body back to start position. Exhale as you push up.

Push-up

Target Muscles:
*chest, triceps,
anterior deltoid*

With toes on the floor and
hands wider than shoulder
width apart, lower chest
toward the floor, stopping
when elbows reach a 90-
degree angle. Keep shoulder
blades back and down,
maintain a neutral pelvis by
squeezing glutes and pulling
navel in. Keeping elbows
out, hold, then push from
chest to bring body back to
start position.

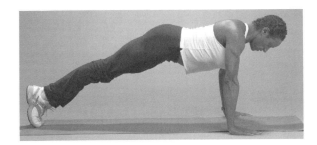

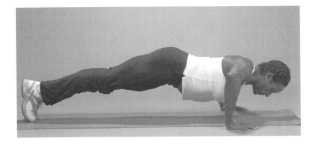

Dumbbell Chest Press

Target Muscles:
chest, triceps, shoulders

Keep knees bent and shoulder
blades together. Start with
weight above your shoulders.
Lower the weight slowly,
keeping hands directly above
your elbows until they form a
90-degree angle from the
shoulder joint. (Do not let
elbows go below shoulders.)
As you push the weight up,
drive your elbows in, squeezing
your chest muscles.

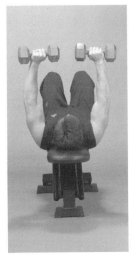
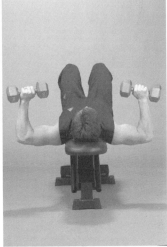

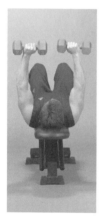
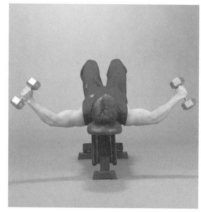

Dumbbell Fly

Target Muscles:
chest, anterior deltoid

Keep knees bent and shoulder blades together. Lower the weight slowly, keeping elbows slightly bent until they are aligned with the shoulder joint. Squeeze the chest muscles as you bring the weight up.

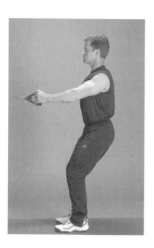
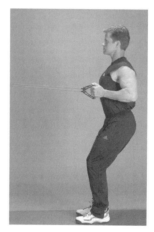

Standing Tubing Row

Target Muscles:
latissimus, trapezius, rhomboids, biceps

Attach tube to a fixed object. In ideal posture, keep thumbs up and shoulder blades down and in. Squeezing elbows tight to the body, pull back until even to midline of the body. The movement will feel like you are folding your back in half. Keep your glutes tight, rib cage up, and navel pulled up and in. You may wish to double up the bands to increase the intensity.

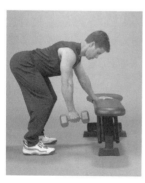
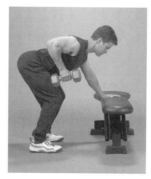

Dumbbell Row

Target Muscles:
latissimus , trapezius, rhomboids, biceps

With one hand placed on bench, slightly bend your knees, flatten your back, squeeze your glutes and pull navel in. Pull shoulder blades back and down, keeping a flat back. While squeezing elbow tight to the body, raise weight until elbow reaches midline. Keep shoulders even. Repeat on opposite side.

Tubing Wide Pull

Target Muscles:
rear deltoids, trapezius, rhomboids

Maintain ideal posture position. With arms straight, shoulder blades down and back, pull tubing across chest until body forms a "T". Keep tension in tubing and wrists straight. Keep rib cage up and pull navel up and in. To increase intensity bring hands closer together to start or change color of tubing. (Great exercise to work those posture muscles.)

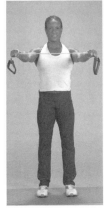 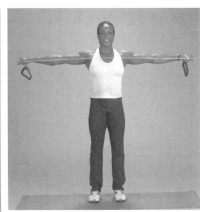

Thoracic Extension

Target Muscles:
lower trapezius, erector spinae

Maintaining ideal posture, raise straight arms overhead, while keeping chest up and shoulders back and down. Try this exercise against the wall with no weights or tubing to start. To avoid arching your back, keep your glutes tight, pull navel up and in. To increase intensity, hold movement at the top for 5–30 seconds. (A great exercise to enhance shoulder strength and range of motion.)

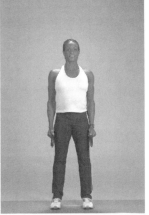 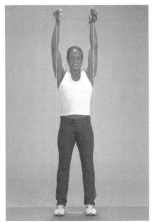

Tubing Shoulder Press

Target Muscles:
anterior deltoid, triceps

Maintain ideal posture with tubing underneath feet and behind elbows, arms extended overhead, chest up and shoulders back and down. Do not arch back; keep glutes tight and navel pulled up and in. Lower elbows until they align with shoulders. Keep hands directly over elbows. This exercise can be more demanding on the shoulder joint, so start slowly with very little resistance.

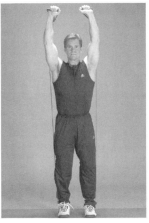 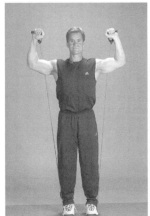

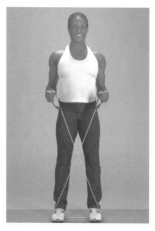 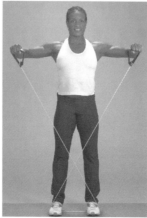

Tubing Lateral Raise

Target Muscles:
medial deltoid,
upper trapezius

In ideal posture position, place tubing under your feet and cross tubing, elbows at your side in a 90-degree angle. Keeping your chest up and shoulders back and down, with the tubing handle in hands, raise elbows to shoulder height keeping arms at 90 degrees. At the top position, the hands, elbows and shoulders should be flat (imagine balancing a cup of water on each joint).

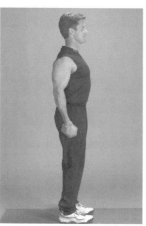 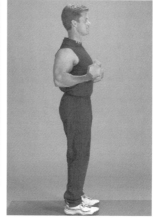

Biceps Curl

Target Muscles:
biceps, forearms,
upper back

Maintaining ideal posture, stand on the tubing or hold dumbbells with palms up. Keep elbows back, raise hands up to chest height only, and keep wrists firm. Squeeze biceps at the top and lower slowly. To increase the forearm muscle involvement, turn hand so the thumb is pointing up (hammer curls).

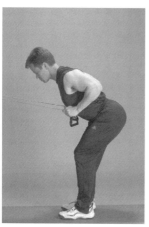 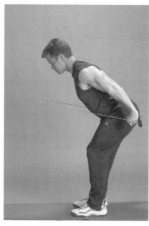

Triceps Kickbacks

Target Muscles:
triceps

Attach tubing to a fixed object. Lean upper body forward 45 degrees, flat back, shoulder blades together, glutes tight, navel pulled up and in, elbows anchored at your side. Hold the tube handles and extend and flex arms back in a slow and controlled movement. Shoulders, elbows and wrists should be aligned at end of movement. This exercise can also be performed with dumbbells.

Triceps Extensions

Target Muscles:
triceps

Lying on bench with chest up, shoulders back and down, raise arms above head,. With weights in hands, slowly flex elbows bringing the weights toward your head. Slowly extend the arms back up. Keep elbows pointed toward the ceiling.

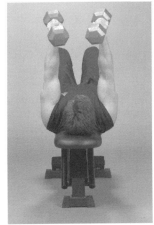 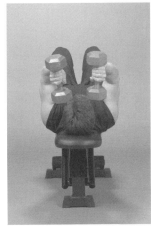

Triceps Dip

Target Muscles:
triceps, shoulders

This is a more advanced movement as it places more stress on the shoulder joint. Use a fixed chair or bench. Bend knees, keep chest up, pull navel up and in as you lower your body. Pivot at your elbows only.

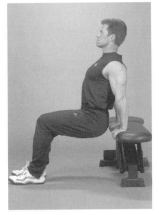 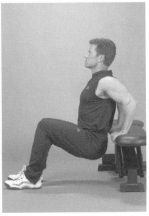

Forearms

Target Muscles:
forearms

While kneeling, rest elbows on the bench. Maintain neutral alignment (pelvic tilt, navel in, shoulders retracted). Raise and lower weights by moving wrists. All forearm movements also work well with rubber tubing.

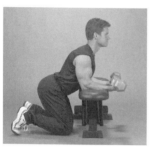 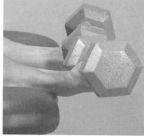

Flexion
With palms up, slowly curl weight up.

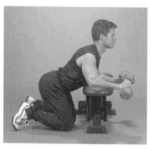 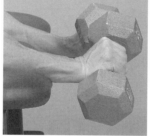

Extension
With palms down, using less weight, slowly bring knuckles up.

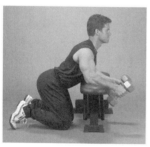 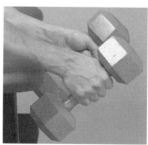

Ulna Deviation
With thumbs up, use the same amount of weight as with extensions. Raise thumb side of hand up and down.

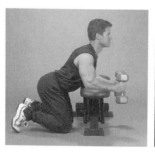 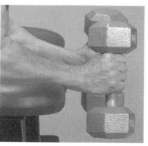

Rotation
Use the same amount of weight as with extension and deviation. Slowly rotate weight in and out.

Strength Training Core

Ab Crunch

Target Muscles:

core

Place your fingertips lightly on your thighs. Keep your glutes tight and pull navel up and in throughout the entire movement. Slowly lift your chest up, reaching your fingertips to your knees. Keep your eyes looking to the ceiling. Exhale during exertion (when coming up). Maintain adequate space between chest and chin.

Progress to an advanced Ab Crunch by crossing one hand to the opposite knee (creating rotation) as you come up. Alternate crossing hand.

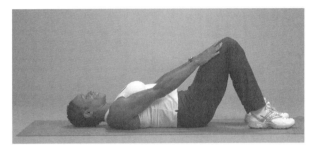

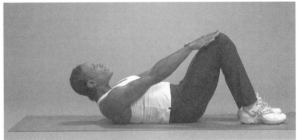

Hip Curl

Target Muscles:

core

Lying on your back, arms overhead holding on to fixed object, try to keep arms straight and shoulder blades down and in, knees together, heels close to your glutes. Pull navel up and in and slowly pull your knees into your chest. Do not lower knees past the hips. When you first begin, your range of motion may be small. As you get stronger, this will slowly improve. (A great exercise for core strength and lower back flexibility.)

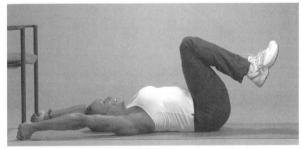

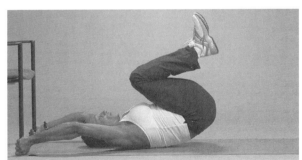

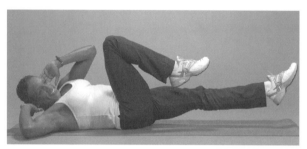

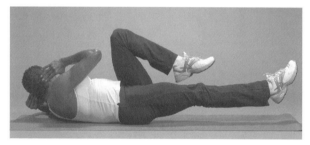

Bicycle

Target Muscles:
core

Lie on floor with shoulder blades retracted, navel pulled up and in, glutes tight. With both legs raised slightly, bring one knee toward midline while bringing opposite elbow toward knee. Alternate knees. To make the exercise easier, keep the heel of the straightened leg touching the floor.

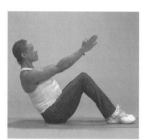

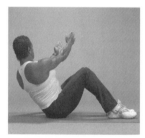

Seated Twist

Target Muscles:
core

Start in a seated position with knees bent. Lean back, keep rib cage up, navel pulled up and in, and feet touching the floor. Extend arms with hands apart, slowly twisting side to side while maintaining ideal posture.

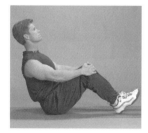

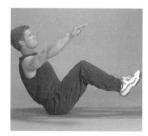

Yoga Crunch

Target Muscles:
core

This is an advanced exercise and is difficult to execute correctly. Start in a seated position with knees bent, hands on knees. Lean back. Slowly raise feet off ground and hands off knees, while balancing on hip bones. Keep your rib cage up, pull navel up and in. Do not round the back. Hold movement for 10–30 seconds.

Back Extension

Target Muscles:
lower and upper back

Lie face down, extend arms at your side, palms facing down, and legs straight. Contract glutes and pull navel up and in. Lift chest off the floor, keeping head in neutral position. Keep the chin pulled in gently. Hold movement for 5–10 seconds.

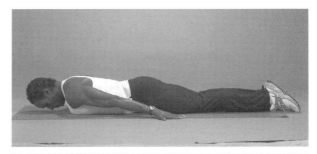

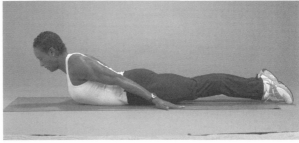

Spinal Balance

Target Muscles:
back, core, shoulders, glutes

On hands and knees, extend one arm forward and lift the opposite leg backward until arm, leg, and core form a straight line. Contract glutes and pull navel up and in. Hold for 5–10 seconds. Repeat on opposite side.

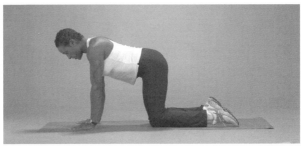

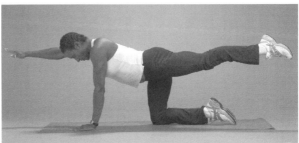

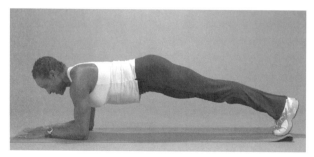

Plank

Target Muscles:
core, shoulders, legs
Position body with toes on
floor, resting on elbows and
hands. Hold body in straight
alignment by tightening glutes
and pull navel up and in.
Hold movement for 5–30
seconds. (A great exercise for
conditioning the entire core.)

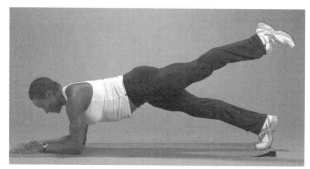

Advanced Plank

Target Muscles:
core, shoulders, legs
Begin in plank position. Slowly
raise one leg off floor, maintaining
balance and tight glutes with
navel pulled up and in. Keep hips
square and hold movement. Hold
movement for 5–30 seconds.
Alternate legs.

Modified Side Plank

Target Muscles:
core, shoulders, hips
Place hand directly under shoulder. Place weight evenly between hand, knee and foot. Raise hips high. Hold 5–30 seconds. Repeat on opposite side.

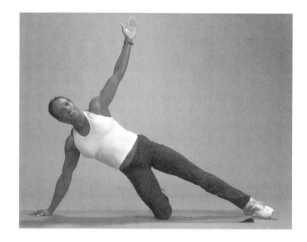

Side Plank

Target Muscles:
core, shoulders, hips
Balance on hand and side of foot, hips high. Maintain strong core with feet together. Hold 5–30 seconds. Repeat on opposite side.

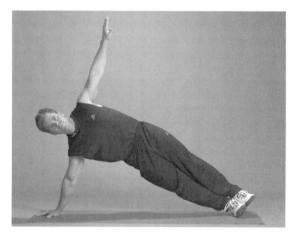

Advanced Side Plank

Target Muscles:
core, shoulders, hips
From side plank position, raise top leg. Hold 5–30 seconds. Repeat on opposite side.

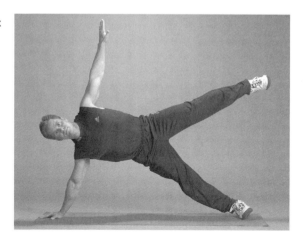

Balance Poses

I have picked two yoga balance poses. They are challenging, but can be great for improving your balance, flexibility and strength. Start these exercises slowly and hold each movement for 10–30 seconds. Try to perfect your technique. These exercises may be done daily. Keep your breathing slow and relaxed.

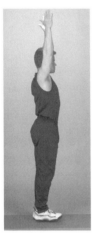
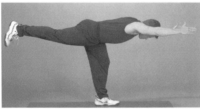
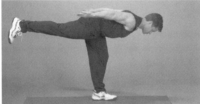

Warrior III

Target Muscles:
quads, glutes, feet, shoulders, back, hamstrings, core

Begin in ideal posture position with arms raised overhead. Slowly bend at waist while lifting one leg backward to form a "T." Arms may stay extended or at your side. Contract glutes and pull navel up and in. Hold movement for 10–30 seconds. Repeat on opposite side.

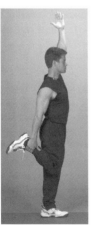
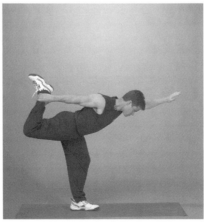

Dancer

Target Muscles:
quads, glutes, feet, shoulders, back, hamstrings, core

Grab ankle or top of foot with one arm and extend the other arm overhead. Slowly bend at waist. Keep knee of stabilizing leg slightly bent. Try to pull the foot away from your glute. Contract glutes, pull navel up and in. Hold movement for 10–30 seconds. Repeat on opposite side.

Stretching/Flexibility

The benefits of stretching are many, from decreasing stress to improving muscle imbalances. Stretching exercises should be performed after the body is warmed up or at the end of your exercise program. There are virtually hundreds of different stretching exercises from which to choose. I have chosen very basic stretches that cover the entire body. Don't neglect the stretching portion of your exercise program. Start with just a few stretching exercises and gradually build from there. Focus on proper body alignment and breathing (deep, slow breathing). Stretching exercises may be done daily. A few general rules apply to stretching:

- hold each stretch 10–60 seconds;
- maintain ideal posture throughout all stretches; and,
- do not stretch to a point of discomfort.

Big 3 Tubing Stretch

Target Muscles:
hamstrings, adductors, hips, lower back

Lying on your back, place tubing or towel around your shoe. Keeping one leg straight and touching the floor, bring the other leg straight up, then to your side and finally, across your body. Maintain a slight bend in the knees for all three stretches. Repeat with the opposite leg (three stretches each leg).

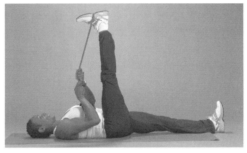

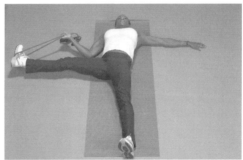

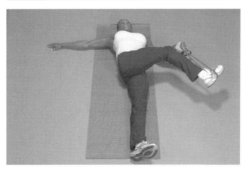

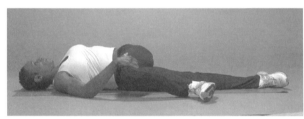

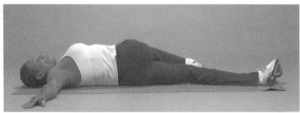

Hip Stretch

Target Muscles:
hips, lower back

Lying on your back, keep right leg straight. Lift left leg over the right hip. Place your right hand on your left knee and pull knee gently in and hold stretch. Keep both shoulders flat against the floor. Repeat on opposite side.

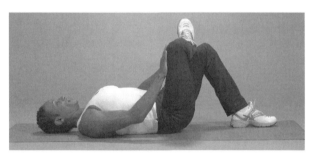

Piriformis I (Beginner)

Target Muscles:
hips, piriformis

On your back, cross ankle over opposite knee. Gently push knee away from your upper body with your hand. To increase the intensity of this stretch, sit up with your back against a wall. Repeat on opposite side.

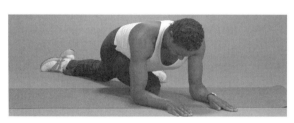

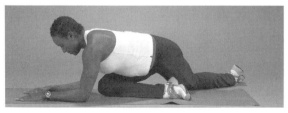

Piriformis II (Advanced)

Target Muscles:
hips, piriformis

This stretch may be difficult to perform if you have knee problems. On left knee, bring the right knee under the body and slowly cross over to the left shoulder. Gently lower your upper body to your knee. Repeat on opposite side.

Child's Pose

Target Muscles:
back, shoulders, lats

From hands and knees, push hips back toward the heels. Keep arms straight, reaching forward. To stretch out your lats, reach to the side. (A great relaxation stretch.)

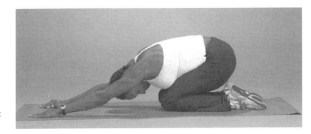

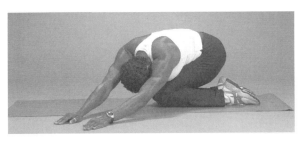

Frog Stretch

Target Muscles:
adductors, hips, back

Resting on knees and forearms, spread legs apart, chest up, flat back. To increase stretch, move hips slowly back.

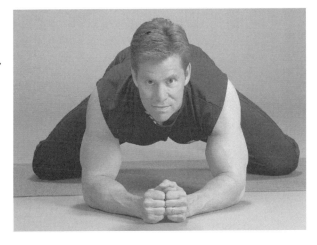

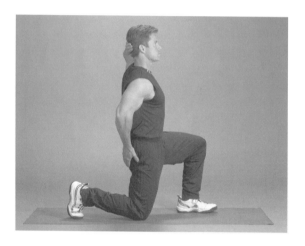

Kneeling Hip Flexor

Target Muscles:
hip flexors, quadriceps

On right knee, place right hand on right glute. Place left hand behind your head, pull elbow back to open up the rib cage. Contract glutes and pull navel up and in. Try to pull your right knee forward (isometrically) without changing your pelvic tilt. Repeat on the opposite side. (A great stretch for runners and golfers.)

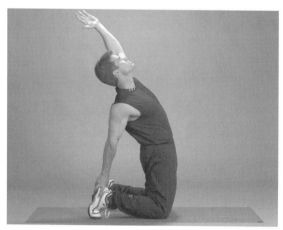

Modified Camel

Target Muscles:
quadriceps, hip flexors, shoulders, core, neck

From kneeling position, place right hand on right heel and raise left hand overhead. Squeeze your glutes to protect your lower back. As you reach up and back with your left hand, try to push the hips forward, squeezing the glutes and pulling your navel into your spine. Repeat on opposite side.

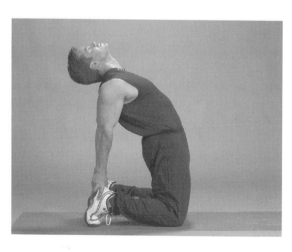

Camel

Target Muscles:
quadriceps, hip flexors, shoulders, core, neck

As you become comfortable with the modified camel, try this regular camel stretch. From kneeling position, place hands on heels. Gently press the hips forward and lift the chest to the sky. Tighten your glutes and pull your navel into your spine.

Advanced Hamstring Stretch

Target Muscles:
hamstrings, glutes

Kneel on left knee and move right foot forward with right knee slightly bent. Place hands on floor on either side of the right leg to support your posture and slide your right leg forward until your left thigh is in line with your back (on a diagonal to the floor).

Keep chest up and maintain a flat back. Pull navel up and in. Raise toes of right foot toward the ceiling and straighten right knee for one second. Lower toes. Then bend right knee again and hold 15–30 seconds. Repeat 2 or 3 times on each side.

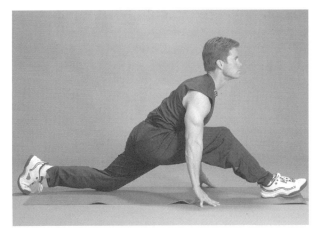

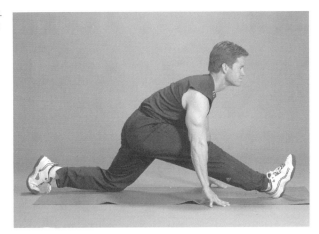

Overhead Reach

Target Muscles:
lower back

In ideal posture position, keep shoulders back and down and chest up. Extend arms overhead, clasp right hand on left wrist. Gently pull left arm up and over to the right side. Repeat on the opposite side.

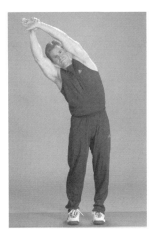

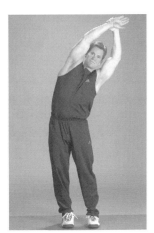

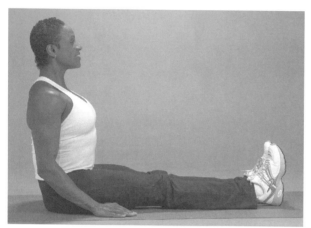

Back Stretch

Target Muscles:
neck, upper and lower back, hamstrings, calves
Scoot back against the wall, allowing the sitting bones to press firmly into the floor, legs forward on floor. Take a deep breath in and exhale as you tuck your chin, pull your navel into your spine and slowly walk your hands forward as you bend at the waist. Slowly raise back up and repeat stretch 2–4 times.

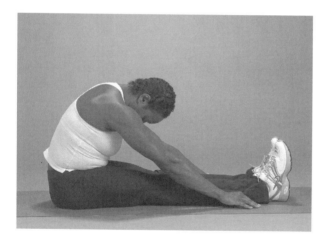

Neck Stretch
(Lateral Flexion)

Target Muscles:
neck, trapezius

With back against the wall, keep shoulders pulled back and down and hands on floor. Tip head to side taking ear directly to shoulder. Reach hand out to your side, away from the head. Hold stretch 10–30 seconds on each side.

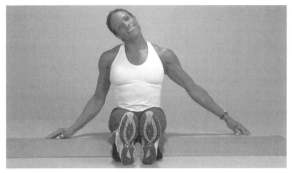

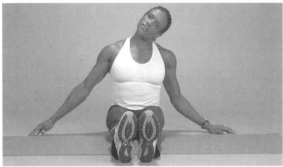

Neck Stretch
(Rotation)

Target Muscles:
neck, trapezius

Keep shoulders pulled back and down and hands on floor. Rotate head slowly side to side, looking in opposite directions. Hold stretch 10–30 seconds on each side.

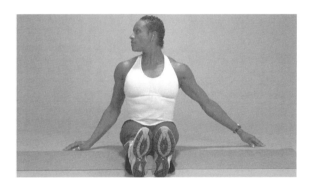

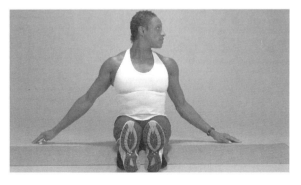

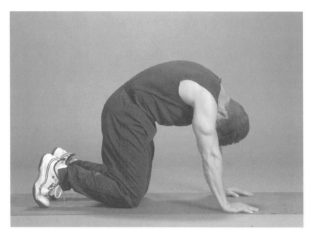

Cat and Dog

Target Muscles:
back, core, shoulders, neck

On hands and knees, round your spine (cat position). Pull your navel into your spine. In the dog position, bring your head up, pull your shoulders back and down and rotate pelvic positions so that back assumes a "U" shape. In both movements, keep your arms slightly bent and knees bent at 90-degree angle.

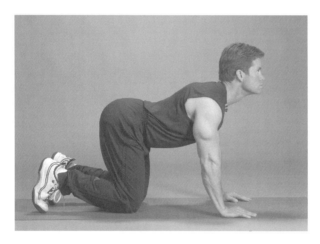

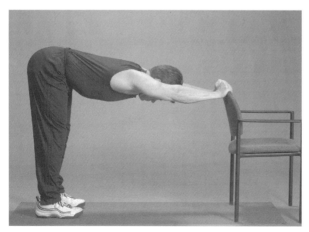

Modified Downward Dog

Target Muscles:
full body

Hold onto a fixed object, feet shoulder-width apart. Push hips back and push shoulders toward floor. Keep back, head and arms in neutral alignment. Modify stretch by slightly bending knees. (A great stretch that is easy to perform and can be done virtually anywhere.)

Modified Upward Dog

Target Muscles:
full body

With feet shoulder-width apart, place hands on fixed object, face forward, chest up, glutes tight, pull navel up and in. Slowly pull hips forward, head back, shoulders down and in.

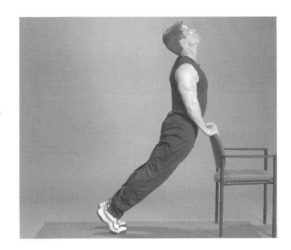

Downward Dog

Target Muscles:
full body

Keep hands slightly wider than shoulder width, fingers spread apart, wrists neutral (flat). Push hips toward ceiling and push chest toward your thighs, knees slightly bent. As you become warmed up, straighten legs more and slowly lower heels to the floor, pull navel up and in. Hold stretch 10–30 seconds, repeat 2 or 3 times.

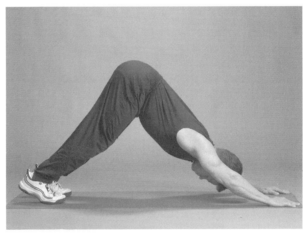

Upward Dog

Target Muscles:
full body

Place hands directly under shoulders. From the downward dog position, slowly lower your hips, pull toes underneath, squeeze your glutes, pull head up and shoulders back and down.
In both movements, keep your arms slightly bent. Pull navel up and in. Keep knees slightly off the floor. Hold stretch 10–30 seconds, repeat 2 or 3 times.

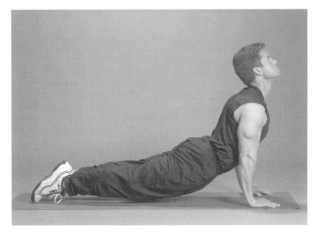

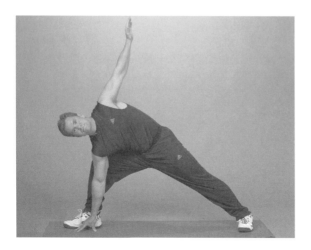

Yoga Extended Angle

Target Muscles:
adductors, quadriceps, glutes, shoulders, back, core
Square up front foot, align knee over the second toe, back foot turned in 3–4 inches. Lunge forward, keeping the weight centered over the front foot and on the outside of the back foot. Reaching forward, place hand on your knee or at the base of the foot on the floor. Reach up with opposite arm and open up shoulders and chest. Squeeze glutes and pull navel up and in. Repeat on opposite side. (A great rotational stretch, especially for those who play golf, tennis, racquetball, squash or handball.)

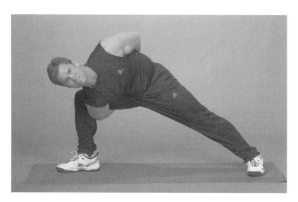

Extended Angle with Shoulder Opener

Target Muscles:
adductors, quadriceps, glutes, shoulders, back, core
This is a more advanced version of the Yoga Extended Angle exercise. Start from the extended angle pose. Bring right arm underneath right leg, keeping shoulders back, then bring left arm around back. Clasp hands together and keep shoulders open. Maintain your lunge posture. Repeat on opposite side.

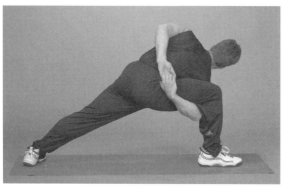

Sample Exercise Programs

I have designed a few sample exercise routines for the beginner, intermediate, and advanced exerciser. The goal with all exercises is to challenge the body while maintaining ideal posture and good technique throughout each exercise. Start slowly and listen to your body.

Beginner

Posture Focus on getting into ideal posture alignment. Line up the toes, keep knees slightly bent, hips neutral, chest up, shoulders back and down, and head centered over the body.

Dynamic Warm-Up Spend a few minutes getting your body warmed-up with dynamic stretches. Use slow and controlled movements. Get into a habit of warming your body up for 3–5 minutes before you exercise.

Cardiovascular Exercise Exercise for 5–15 minutes, at an easy intensity level, 2–4 times per week. Maintain ideal posture throughout your Cardiovascular Exercise session.

Strength Training The exercises here cover the large muscle groups. Focus on perfect technique with 1 or 2 sets per exercise of 4–10 reps per set, 2 or 3 times per week.

Recommended Exercises	Page
Chair Squat	127
Straight Leg "Yoga" Lunge	128
Tubing Wide Pull	133
–or– Standing Tubing Row	132
Back Extension	139
Ab Crunch	137

Stretching

Recommended Exercises	Page
Cat and Dog	150
Big 3 Tubing Stretch	143

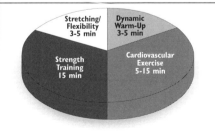

Beginning Exercise Program 35–40 minutes 2 or 3 times per week

Intermediate

Posture

Dynamic Warm-Up 5 minutes.

Cardiovascular Exercise Work for 15–20 minutes, 2–4 times per week.
Start adding interval training (higher-intensity bursts between recovery periods).
Maintain ideal posture throughout your Cardiovascular Exercise session.

Strength Training Attempt 2 or 3 sets per exercise, 8–12 reps per set,
2 or 4 times per week. You may want to split up your strength training routine
(upper body Monday and Thursday, lower body and core Tuesday and Friday).
Maintain ideal posture and technique with each exercise.

Recommended Exercises	Page
Lower Body	
Chair or Dumbbell Squats—Hold each exercise for 3–5 seconds at the bottom of the movement, maintaining perfect alignment.	127
Stride Lunge—4–6 reps per set, hold each exercise for 2–5 seconds at the bottom of the movement	128
Tubing Side Step—Ideal posture, use green tubing, go slow and feel the hips and legs working.	129

Recommended Exercises	Page
Upper Body	
Push-up –or– Modified Push-up	130-131
Standing Tubing or Dumbbell Rows	132
Thoracic Extension—No weight, hold movement at the top	133
Biceps Curl	134

Recommended Exercises	Page
Core	
Hip Curl	137
Modified Side Plank	141
Spinal Balance	139

Stretching:

	Page
Downward and Upward Dog	151
Hip Stretch	144
Kneeling Hip Flexor	146

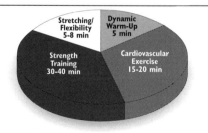

Stretching/ Flexibility 5-8 min
Dynamic Warm-Up 5 min
Strength Training 30-40 min
Cardiovascular Exercise 15-20 min

Intermediate Exercise Program 60–70 minutes 2 or 4 times per week

I have split the advanced exercise routine into two different workouts. Each workout may be completed 1 or 2 times per week. Remember to incorporate rest and recovery in your weekly program.

Advanced

Workout #1—Monday/Thursday

Posture

Dynamic Warm-Up 5 minutes

Cardiovascular Exercise 15–20 minutes of steady state (maintaining the same intensity) exercise, moderate to high intensity.

Strength Training

Recommended Exercises	Page
Lower Body	
Dumbbell Squat—3 or 4 sets, 8–12 reps per set.	127
Straight Leg "Yoga" Lunge—3 sets; hold each exercise for 20–30 seconds. Don't forget to breathe.	128
Stride Lunge—3 or 4 sets, 4–6 reps; hold each exercise for 5 seconds at the bottom of the movement.	128
Tubing Side Step—Maintain ideal posture. Use green or red tubing.	129
Single Leg Calf Raise: 3 sets of 8–12 reps; hold exercise for 1–2 seconds at the top of the movement. Maintain ideal posture.	129
Core	
Side Plank—Hold movement for 15–30 seconds.	141
Yoga Crunch—Hold movement for 10-20 seconds; maintain ideal posture.	138
Hip Curl—6–10 reps, slowly.	137
Balance Poses	
Warrior III—Hold for 20–30 seconds, 1 or 2 sets	142
Stretching Hold each movement for 10–30 seconds, repeat 2 times.	
Downward and Upward Dog	151
Modified Camel	146
Yoga Extended Angle	152

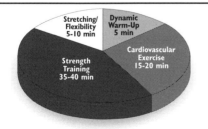

Advanced Exercise Program 65-75 minutes 1 or 2 times per week

Workout #2—Tuesday/Friday

Posture

Dynamic Warm-Up 5 minutes

Cardiovascular Exercise 15–20 minutes of interval training, moderate to high intensity.

Strength Training

Balance

Stretching Hold each movement for 10–30 seconds, repeat 2 times.

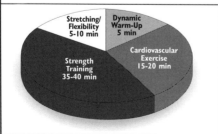

Advanced Exercise Program 65-75 minutes 1 or 2 times per week

EXERCISE LOG

WEEK OF ___ / ___ / ___

	Warm-Up Stretching	Cardiovascular Exercise	Strength Training	Balance / Flexibility	Daily Physical Activity	Comments
MON	5 min.	Elliptical Training (high intensity) [15]	Lower Body Core [35]	Balance: 2 min. Flexibility: 5 min.		Worked on posture with all exercises
TUE	5 min.	Treadmill walking (moderate intensity) [20]	Chest Back [30]	Flexibility: 5 min.	15 min. walk after dinner	Focused on techniques and strength training
WED	5 min. before yoga class				Power Yoga class 60 min.	Breathing significantly better Great Class!
THU	5 min.	Stairclimbers (high intensity) [15]	Shoulders Arms Core [30]	Balance: 3 min. Flexibility: 5 min.		High energy Felt strong
FRI	5 min.	Stationary Bike (moderate intensity) [20]	Lower Body Core [35]	Flexibility: 8 min.		Working on better alignment and lower body
SAT	5 min.	Played Tennis [90]		Flexibility: 8 min. after tennis		Backhand needs work!
SUN	10 min. before golf				walked 18 holes of golf	Felt great after walking the 18

Frequently Asked Exercise Questions

1. If exercise is so good for us, then why don't people do it?

First, people feel they just don't have time to exercise. In reality, you cannot afford not to exercise. Plan exercise into your schedule and make it a priority. Second, exercise needs to be fun and enjoyable. Experiment with your exercise program and try to include activities you enjoy.

2. How much exercise is enough?

This depends on your personal goals. If you want to achieve a very high fitness level, then the time needed for exercise will be greater than someone who wants to develop basic conditioning. One of the magical things about the human body is that it gets better with use. You do not have to spend a lot of time to keep your body in good condition. Small doses of exercise on a consistent basis are very beneficial. Developing consistent exercise habits will give you the greatest long-term benefits. Start slowly with your program and begin to develop good exercise patterns.

3. Do I need to buy special exercise machines and equipment to get a good workout?

Not at all. The only exercise tool that is necessary is your own body. You may want to supplement your program with other equipment, but it is not necessary.

4. Is it expensive to start an exercise program?

No. If you would like to get started in your own home, you can start without spending any money. Or, you may elect to outfit your home with some exercise equipment at a very low cost.

5. How should I breathe when exercising?

Never hold your breath during exercise. Holding your breath during exercise may increase your blood pressure. When strength training, exhale during *exertion.*

6. Does exercise have to be painful to get results?

You may experience some discomfort when exercising. For instance, you may be out of breath or feel some burning in your muscles. If you are experiencing true pain, your body is signaling you to slow down or to stop. Exercise should not be painful to perform. It may become difficult at times, but should never be painful.

7. Can exercise be fun and enjoyable?

Fitness professionals agree that for people to stay with any exercise program, it *must* be fun and enjoyable. Use exercises you enjoy, not just exercises you think are good for you.

8. **When is the best time to exercise?**

   For most people, the core temperature of the body reaches its peak during the late afternoon and early evening. This is the easiest time for the body to perform at its best. Many people, however, exercise when it fits into their schedules. Depending on your goals, schedule time for your exercise program that fits best for you and stick with it. Make an appointment with yourself for exercise.

9. **Should I eat before I exercise?**

   If you are exercising first thing in the morning, you may want to eat after you exercise. A small balanced snack or meal approximately 1-1/2 hours prior to and after exercise is recommended. If you find you don't have much energy for exercise, focus on eating better, develop good sleep habits and set a goal for balance in your current lifestyle.

10. **What causes muscle soreness and what should I do about it?**

    Muscle soreness is caused by micro-tears in the muscle. Most muscle soreness reaches its peak 48 hours after exercise (commonly referred to as *delayed onset muscle soreness*). Activity that overloads muscle in ways it is not accustomed to can cause muscle soreness.

11. **Is muscle soreness good?**

    It depends on how severe the soreness is. If you are so sore you can hardly walk, this is an indication that your activity level was too severe, and that your progression into the activity was too quick. A small amount of muscle soreness can be beneficial. This slight soreness is an indication that your activity is progressing in the right direction. You are achieving a training effect.

    Active rest, such as walking, stretching or easy swimming, using a sauna or hot tub or getting a massage are excellent ways to help recover from muscle soreness. Remember to enjoy your fitness program and make gradual, yet continual improvements.

12. **How important is rest and recovery?**

    Adequate rest and recovery times are essential for good, long-term health and fitness. Give each muscle group a day off in between workouts to allow the muscle fibers to rebuild. To perform at your optimal level, you need adequate sleep, relaxation time, active rest and good nutrition. If you do not allow for adequate rest and recovery, your potential for injury and burnout increases.

13. **Should I exercise every day?**

    Moving the body on a regular basis is an important ingredient in keeping the body healthy. Strength training can put great demands on the body. Adequate recovery between strength training sessions is important for achieving the greatest benefits. One or two days of rest between strength training workouts is recommended. Cardiovascular and flexibility training can be done daily. Start slowly. Listen to your body and take days off as needed.

Exercise Considerations

1. You may wish to consult your physician or exercise professional before you begin your exercise program. I highly recommend hiring a *qualified personal trainer* for three to five sessions to get you started on the right track.

2. Make sure you are well-hydrated before, during and after exercise.

3. Exercise greatly increases body temperature. Be careful when exercising in a warm environment.

4. Wear comfortable, breathable clothing and a good pair of shoes when exercising.

Chapter 23

Meal Patterning Recipes

Shoot for the moon. Even if you miss it,
you will land among the stars.

— Les Brown

The recipes in this section introduce some healthy alternatives to traditional ingredients. Some of these recipes are original and others are adaptations. Use these recipes as a start, then experiment with your own favorites to convert them into more healthy versions.

Don't forget, food preparation does not have to be complicated. Steamed vegetables drizzled with olive oil or low-fat cottage cheese with fresh fruit are simple and wonderful. A turkey sandwich on whole grain bread with mustard, lettuce, and tomatoes is still very healthy for lunch.

Enjoy these recipe ideas, and then let your imagination fly!

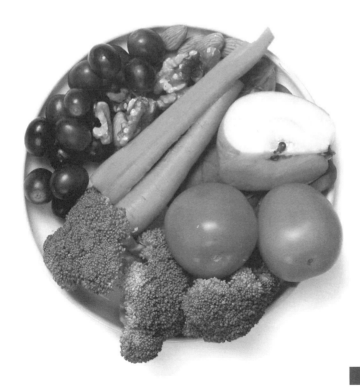

Index of Recipes

Breakfast

Oatmeal on the Run
Makes 1 serving
1/2 to 2/3 cup rolled oats
1-1/2 tbs. fruit (raisins, dried cherries, blueberries or strawberries)
1 to 1-1/2 tbs. slivered almonds, walnuts, flaxmeal or flaxseed oil
1/2 to 2/3 cup soy or skim milk
1/2 scoop soy or whey protein powder (optional)

Place all ingredients in a small bowl with lid. Let stand in refrigerator overnight or 10 minutes prior to eating. No cooking required. Fast, easy, healthy and tastes great.

Calories: 387, CHO: 50g, FAT: 11g, PRO: 22g

Oatmeal Plus
Makes 1 serving
2/3 cup rolled oats
1/2 scoop soy or whey protein powder
1 tsp. cinnamon
1-1/2 tbs. dried fruit
1 tbs. walnuts, almonds, flaxmeal or flaxseed oil
1-1/4 cups water
1 tsp. vanilla
1/2 to 2/3 cup soy or skim milk

In a saucepan, mix well water and protein powder. Add the oats and bring to a boil, stirring occasionally. When mixture starts to thicken, cover the pot and turn off the heat. Let stand for 10 minutes and add the remaining ingredients. Mix well and serve.

Calories: 388, CHO: 48g, FAT: 12g, PRO: 22g

Heart Healthy Granola
Makes 14 1/2-cup servings
6 cups rolled oats
2 tbs. expeller pressed canola oil
1 cup dried fruit (raisins, cherries, cranberries)
1-1/2 cups dried apples, chopped into small pieces
1/3 cup ground flaxseeds or walnuts
2 tbs. brown sugar or Stevia Plus equivalent

Preheat oven to 350°. Mix all ingredients except the dried fruit in a large bowl. Spread evenly in a shallow baking pan and bake for 15 minutes. Remove from oven and stir so granola will cook uniformly. Continue to bake 10 to 15 minutes until golden. Remove from oven and mix in dried fruit. Cool and store in a covered container. Add 1/2 cup skim or soy milk to granola (optional). Your kids will love this for breakfast and snacks.

Calories: 292, CHO: 47g, FAT: 8g, PRO: 8g [excluding milk]

Egg White Omelet

Makes 2 servings

8 egg whites (free-range eggs)
2 egg yolks (free-range eggs)
1/2 tbs. extra virgin olive oil
1 tbs. shredded cheddar cheese [low-fat]

1/4 cup onion, sliced or chopped
1/4 cup green or red bell pepper,
  sliced or chopped
1/4 cup mushrooms

In an omelet pan or skillet, sauté vegetables; set aside. Coat skillet with oil. Pour beaten eggs into skillet. As eggs begin to set, lift edges and tilt pan to move uncooked eggs to bottom. Spread cooked vegetables over half the eggs. Sprinkle on cheese. Flip remaining half of eggs over vegetables and cheese. Serve with sliced fruit.

Calories: 196, CHO: 5g, FAT: 12g, PRO: 17g [excluding fruit]

2-Minute Egg Whites

Makes 2 servings

6 egg whites (free-range eggs)
2 egg yolks (free-range eggs)
1/2 tbs. extra virgin olive oil

1/4 cup onion, chopped
1/4 cup green bell pepper, chopped
2 tbs. Summer Salsa (pg. 176) or
  prepared salsa

Coat a microwave-safe bowl with olive oil. Add 6 egg whites and the two yolks. Add chopped onions and green peppers, mixing until blended. Cover with a paper plate and cook in the microwave for 2–3 minutes. Remove from the microwave and top with salsa. Enjoy a low-calorie, energy-boosting breakfast or snack.

Calories: 202, CHO: 10g, FAT: 10g, PRO: 18g

Scrambled Eggs

Makes 2 servings

4 egg whites (free-range eggs)
2 egg yolks (free-range eggs)
1 large garlic clove, pressed
1 tbs. fresh oregano, chopped
1 tbs. grated cheddar cheese (low-fat)

1/2 red bell pepper, diced
1/2 green bell pepper, diced
1/2 small white onion, diced
1/2 tbs. extra virgin olive oil
salt and pepper to taste

Whisk eggs and spices in medium bowl. Stir in peppers and onion. Lightly coat a medium skillet with extra virgin olive oil and heat. Pour egg mixture into skillet. Scramble until cooked. Sprinkle with cheddar cheese.

Calories: 230, CHO: 10g, FAT: 14g, PRO: 16g

Simple Seafood Scramble

Makes 2 servings

6 egg whites (free-range eggs)
2 egg yolks (free-range eggs)
1 large garlic clove, pressed
1 tbs. fresh basil, chopped
1 tsp. fresh dill, chopped
1/2 cup chopped, cooked shrimp, crab
  or scallops (or combination)

1 celery stalk, minced
1/4 cup tomatoes, finely chopped
2 scallions, finely chopped
1/4 cup mushrooms, finely chopped
1 tbs. extra-virgin olive oil
salt and pepper to taste
1 or 2 sprigs fresh parsley, for garnish

Whisk eggs and spices in a small bowl. Stir in chopped vegetables and cooked seafood. Pour extra virgin olive oil into nonstick skillet and heat. Pour egg mixture into the skillet; scramble until cooked. Garnish with fresh parsley.

Calories: 221, CHO: 6g, FAT: 13g, PRO: 20g

Quiche

Makes 2 servings

6 egg whites (free-range eggs)
2 egg yolks (free-range eggs)
1/4 tsp. pepper
1/2 cup sliced mushrooms
1 tbs. expeller pressed canola oil or extra virgin olive oil

1/2 cup chopped broccoli
1 cup skim or soy milk or water
1/2 cup sliced onion

Coat quiche dish with oil. Mix egg whites and yolks with milk and pour into quiche dish. Sauté onion in a small amount of oil until it begins to brown, add green pepper and mushrooms. Sauté until all the water from the mushrooms is gone and the vegetables are soft. Add pepper. Cool slightly and add to egg mixture. Stir to distribute evenly. Bake at 325° for 1 hour or until knife inserted into center comes out clean. Quick Tip: Combine all ingredients, cover with paper towel and cook in microwave oven for 2 1/2 to 3 1/2 minutes, until eggs are thoroughly cooked.

Calories: 263, CHO: 13g, FAT: 15g, PRO: 19

Oatmeal Pancakes

Makes 6-7 servings (approximately 20 pancakes)

1/4 cup soy or skim milk
12 egg whites (free-range eggs)
3 egg yolks (free-range eggs)
1 tbs. extra virgin olive oil or
  expeller pressed canola oil

3 cups rolled oats
1 cup low-fat cottage cheese
1 cup natural applesauce
1 tsp. vanilla
1 tsp. cinnamon

Mix all ingredients except oil in a blender until smooth (add more milk for creamier batter). Place in a large mixing bowl and let stand for five minutes. Add oil to griddle or skillet. Pour 1/3 cup batter per pancake onto hot griddle. Cook until bubbles form, then flip. Add spoon of fruit or natural applesauce for topping.

Per pancake: Calories: 98, CHO: 15g, FAT: 2g, PRO: 5g [excluding fruit topping]

Power Pancakes

Makes 6-7 servings [approximately 20 pancakes]

2 cups whole grain flour
1 tbs. aluminum-free baking powder
10 egg whites (free-range eggs)
2 egg yolks (free-range eggs)
1-1/2 cups sliced strawberries or blueberries
1 cup soy or whey protein powder

1 tbs. brown sugar or Stevia Plus
equivalent
1 banana
2 cups soy milk or skim milk
1-1/2 tsp. expeller pressed canola oil
or extra virgin olive oil

Mix all ingredients except berries. Beat until blended; don't over beat. If mixture is too stiff, add more milk. Fold fruit into batter. Lightly oil non-stick griddle. Pour 1/3 cup batter per pancake onto griddle and cook until bubbles form, then flip.

Tip: Add spoon of fruit or natural applesauce for topping.

Per pancake: Calories: 126, CHO: 16g, FAT: 2g, PRO: 11g [excluding topping]

Waffles and Fruit

Makes 3 servings [6 waffles]

1-1/2 cups whole grain flour
1 tbs. aluminum-free baking powder
2 tsp. honey or Stevia Plus equivalent
3 tbs. expeller pressed canola oil or
extra virgin olive oil

2 free-range eggs
1 cup soy or skim milk
1/2 cup fruit, sliced

In medium bowl, combine milk, oil and honey. Beat well with an electric mixer. In a separate bowl, sift together flour and baking powder. Add dry ingredients to egg mixture and beat well. Add more milk if necessary. Add fruit to batter. Cook in pre-heated waffle iron.

Calories: 226, CHO: 27g, FAT: 10g, PRO: 7g

Blender Breakfast

Makes 2 servings

1/2 cup soy or skim milk
6 oz. tofu, firm
1 scoop soy or whey protein powder
2 cups frozen fruit (strawberries, blueberries, cherries)

2 tbs. flaxseed oil
1 banana
1 tsp. vanilla

Combine all ingredients in blender and mix until smooth.

Calories: 352, CHO: 33g, FAT: 16g, PRO: 19g

Snacks

Energized Bars

Makes approximately 12 2-inch bars (serving size: one bar)

1–20 oz. can crushed pineapple (in own juice)
1/2 cup crushed almonds or walnuts
2 cups rolled oats

3 scoops soy or whey protein powder
1 cup chopped dried fruit
1-1/2 tsp. cinnamon

Combine all ingredients. Spread in 13 x 9 inch pan sprayed with nonstick spray. Bake at 200° for 1-1/2 hours. Cool and slice. Store in refrigerator.

Great snack anytime.

Calories: 200, CHO: 33g, FAT: 4g, PRO: 8g

Potato Chips

Makes 2 servings

1 medium sweet or redskin potato
dash of salt

2 tbs. extra virgin olive oil

Cut potato into 1/8-inch slices. Place sliced potatoes in plastic bag with oil and salt. Shake well. Spread potatoes in a single layer on wax paper. Heat in microwave for 1 minute on high. Flip potatoes and heat for another minute. Flip potatoes a third time and heat for 1 more minute or until slightly crispy.

Calories: 96.5, CHO: 13g, FAT: 4.5g, PRO: 1g

Turkey Roll-Up

Makes 3 roll-ups

3 slices deli turkey
15 almonds or walnuts

1 small apple or kiwi

Chop fruit and nuts. Roll up in turkey.

Calories: 140, CHO: 10g, FAT: 8g, PRO: 7g

Easy Egg Whites

Makes 1 serving

4 egg whites (free-range eggs)
1 egg yolk (free-range eggs)

1/2 tbs. extra virgin olive oil
1-1/2 tbs. Summer Salsa (pg. 176) or
  prepared salsa

Pour oil into microwaveable bowl and tilt to coat sides. Blend eggs and add to prepared bowl. Cover with paper plate or paper towel. Cook for 2 minutes in the microwave on high or until the center is done. Slide egg white onto a plate; top with salsa.

Quick and easy nutritious snack (add fruit or vegetables to make into a meal).

Calories: 170, CHO: 3g, FAT: 10g, PRO: 17g

CJ's Special Smoothie

Makes 3 12 oz. servings

3 cups water
2 scoops soy or whey protein powder
1–16 oz. bag frozen unsweetened berries

1 banana
1-1/2 tbs. flaxseed oil

Combine ingredients in blender. Cover and blend at high speed about 1 minute. Keep refrigerated.

Calories: 194, CHO: 24g, FAT: 6g, PRO: 11g

Strawberry Dream Smoothie

Makes 2 servings

2 cups frozen strawberries
1 cup soy or skim milk
3 tbs. strawberry preserves

2 scoops soy or whey protein powder
1-1/2 tbs. flaxseed oil

Combine ingredients in blender. Cover and blend at high speed about 1 minute.

Calories: 305, CHO: 24g, FAT: 13g, PRO: 23g

KJ's Chocolate Smoothie

Makes 2 servings

1 cup Soy Delicious® Frozen Dessert
(chocolate velvet)
1 cup carob soy milk

2 scoops soy or whey protein powder
2 tbs. whole almonds

Combine ingredients in blender. Cover and blend at high speed about 1 minute. Pour into frosted glasses. Yum!

Calories: 314, CHO: 32g, FAT: 10g, PRO: 24g

Natural Peanut Butter Smoothie

Makes 3 8 oz. servings

1 cup orange juice
1 cup soy or skim milk
2 tbs. natural crunchy peanut butter
2 tbs. flaxseed oil

2 scoops soy or whey protein powder
1/2 tsp. non-alcohol vanilla extract
1 cup ice

Place ingredients in a blender. Blend until rich and creamy.

Calories: 240, CHO: 15g, FAT: 12g, PRO: 18g

Berry Blast Smoothie
Makes 3 12 oz. servings

2 cups water
2 scoops soy or whey protein powder
1/2 cup non-fat plain yogurt

2 tbs. almond butter or whole almonds
1 cup frozen blueberries
1 cup frozen strawberries

Combine all ingredients in blender. Blend until rich and creamy.

Calories: 249, CHO: 17g, FAT: 13g, PRO: 16g

Applesauce Plus
Makes 1 serving

2/3 to 1 cup natural applesauce
1 tbs. dried fruit

1 tbs. walnuts or almonds
1 tbs. soy or whey protein powder

Combine ingredients in a bowl and stir. Great anytime snack to satisfy that sweet tooth (balanced, easy and great tasting).

Calories: 266, CHO: 45g, FAT: 6g, PRO: 8g

Yogurt Crunch
Makes 2 servings

1 cup non-fat plain or vanilla yogurt
3/4 cup fresh blueberries or other fruit
1/4 cup rolled oats

2 tbs. slivered or sliced almonds
1 packet Stevia Plus (optional)

Spoon yogurt into bowl and add Stevia Plus sweetener if desired. Add fruit, then nuts and top with rolled oats. Eat immediately or store in refrigerator. Great for breakfast, lunch or a snack.

Calories: 201, CHO: 28g, FAT: 5g, PRO: 11g

Peach Oat Bran Muffins
Makes 12 muffins

1-1/2 cups oat bran
1/2 cup whole grain flour
2 tsp. aluminum-free baking powder
1/8 tsp. cinnamon
1 cup chopped peaches, pineapple or blueberries

1/3 cup honey
2 tbs. expeller pressed canola oil
2 free-range egg whites
1/4 cup slivered almonds

Preheat oven to 425°. Combine dry ingredients and set aside. In separate bowl, blend liquid ingredients. Pour liquid ingredients over dry ingredients and mix just until blended. Stir in fruit. Coat muffin tin with oil. Pour equal amounts of batter into each of 12 muffin cups. Bake for 18–20 minutes. Allow to cool slightly; remove from muffin tin to cool.

Calories: 150, CHO: 19g, FAT: 6g, PRO: 5g

Flax Bran Muffins

Makes 12 muffins

1-1/2 cups unbleached flour
3/4 cup flax meal
3/4 cup oat bran
2/3 cup brown sugar
2 tsp. baking soda
1 tsp. aluminum-free baking powder
3 free-range egg whites
1/2 tsp. salt

2 tsp. cinnamon
1-1/2 cups carrots, shredded
2 apples, shredded
1/2 cup raisins
3/4 cup walnuts, chopped
3/4 cup soy or skim milk
1 tsp. vanilla

Preheat over to 350°. Combine dry ingredients. Add carrots, apples, raisins and nuts. In a separate bowl, blend liquid ingredients. Pour liquid ingredients over dry. Mix until just combined. Divide mixture into muffin cups. Bake for 20 minutes. Allow to cool slightly; remove from muffin tin to cool.

Calories: 157, CHO: 22g, FAT: 5g, PRO: 6g

Trail Mix

Makes 1 serving

1/3 cup rolled oats
1 tbs. slivered almonds or walnuts
1/8 cup raisins or dried cherries

Mix together and eat as a snack.

To save time, make multiple servings; store in air-tight container.

Calories: 256, CHO: 38g, FAT: 8g, PRO: 8g

Salads

Quinoa Salad
Makes 4 6 oz. servings

1 tsp. lemon juice
1/4 cup extra virgin olive oil
2 tsp. minced cilantro
1/2 tsp. salt
1 cup fresh or frozen corn (liquid reserved)
1/4 cup quinoa, rinsed thoroughly
  (rice, couscous or bulgar may be substituted)

1/4 tsp. cumin seed
1/2 cup canned black beans, rinsed
  and drained
1 medium tomato, diced
1 tbs. red onion, minced

Mix lemon juice, oil, cilantro and salt in small, non-metal bowl; set dressing aside. Bring corn liquid to boil in small saucepan. Add quinoa and cumin; cover and simmer until quinoa absorbs the liquid and is tender, about 10 minutes. Transfer quinoa to a large non-metal bowl; cool slightly. Add corn, remaining ingredients and dressing; toss. Chill and serve.

Calories: 264, CHO: 25g, FAT: 16g, PRO: 5g

Chicken Salad
Makes 4 servings

2 cups steamed chicken or turkey breast, cubed
1 cup sliced green or red grapes
1/2 cup sliced green onion

1/2 cup sliced almonds
2 tbs. canola mayonnaise or plain yogurt

Combine all ingredients and chill. Serve over Romaine lettuce.

Calories: 276, CHO: 14g, FAT: 16g, PRO: 19g

Cherry Chicken Salad
Makes 4 servings

4 chicken breasts, grilled and
cut into 1-inch chunks
1/2 cup dried cherries
1/4 cup light canola salad dressing,
  blended with 1/2 tsp. prepared mustard

1/4 cup broken walnuts
3/4 cup celery, sliced diagonally
1/8 cup onion, chopped

Mix all ingredients. Serve on a bed of greens or as a wrap sandwich.

Calories: 264, CHO: 12g, FAT: 12g, PRO: 27g

Black Bean Mango Salad

Makes 6 servings

2 cans black beans, rinsed and drained
1 can white corn, drained
1/2 green bell pepper, chopped
1/2 red bell pepper, chopped
4 green onions, sliced thin

1 avocado, cubed
1 mango, cubed
2 tbs. extra virgin olive oil
2 tbs. balsamic vinegar

Mix all ingredients. Refrigerate 1 hour. One of my favorites.

Calories: 214, CHO: 32g, FAT: 6g, PRO: 8g

Zesty Three Bean Salad

Makes 10 servings

1–16 oz. can of black beans
1–16 oz. can of navy beans
1–16 oz. can of red beans
2 medium limes, halved
1–12 oz. jar of medium salsa
2 tbs. extra virgin olive oil or expeller pressed canola oil

1-1/2 tbs. chili powder
2 stalks of celery, sliced
1 medium sweet onion, chopped or diced
1 medium tomato, diced

Prepare at least 30 minutes before serving. Drain beans and set aside. In a large bowl, squeeze lime juice. Stir in salsa, oil and chili powder. Mix well. Add drained beans, celery, onion and tomato. Mix. Serve at room temperature. Store in refrigerator.

Stretched recipe: Use 3 large limes, 2 tbs. chili powder, full bottle of salsa, 5 or 6 diced Roma tomatoes and 5 or 6 stalks of celery; substitute 1 large red onion for medium sweet onion. For spicier flavor, add Tabasco to taste or add Cayenne pepper sparingly.

Calories: 173, CHO: 24g, FAT: 5g, PRO: 8g

Salmon Salad

Makes 4 servings

8 tbs. extra virgin olive oil
4 tbs. balsamic vinegar
salt and pepper to taste
1/4 cup vegetable stock or fish broth
4–4 oz. salmon fillets

6 cups spinach or leaf lettuce
2 tbs. capers, drained
1/2 small red onion, thinly sliced
4 tbs. cooked corn kernels

Whisk 6 tablespoons oil and 3 tablespoons vinegar in a small bowl. Season with salt and pepper and set dressing aside. Place remaining oil and vinegar in a large sauté pan; add the broth. Heat to a boil, then reduce temperature and add the salmon. Poach for 15 to 20 minutes, then transfer to a plate and allow to cool. Prepare each serving plate with 1-1/2 cups greens. Add salmon fillet and garnish with capers, red onion and corn. Drizzle balsamic vinaigrette over each serving.

Calories: 346, CHO: 18g, FAT: 18g, PRO: 28g

CJ's Big Salad

Makes 1 serving

1 tbs. balsamic vinegar
1 tbs. extra virgin olive oil
1/2 cup broccoli slaw
5 grape tomatoes
1-1/2 to 2 cups spinach or Romaine lettuce, torn

1/8 cup red peppers, sliced
1 tbs. raisins
1/2 tbs. slivered almonds or walnuts
1–6 oz. can albacore tuna in water

Mix vinegar and oil together; set aside. Mix all other ingredients in large bowl. Drizzle vinegar and oil mixture over top of salad; toss.

This is my lunch 2 or 3 times per week; fast, easy, healthy and I love the taste.

Calories: 367, CHO: 24g, FAT: 19g, PRO: 25g

Citrus Salad

Makes 4–6 servings

1 head red lettuce, torn
1 head Bibb or butter lettuce, torn
1/2 cup chopped celery
2 cans (2 cups) mandarin oranges, drained
1/2 cup chopped almonds, walnuts, pecans or pine nuts

1/3 cup chopped green onion
1/2 cup watercress sprigs, chopped
1/4 cup chopped parsley

Mix together. Toss with Citrus Salad Dressing (see recipe, next page).

Variation: substitute grapefruit sections or diced or sliced avocado for oranges.

Calories: 147, CHO: 16g, FAT: 7g, PRO: 5g

Dressings/Dips

Citrus Salad Dressing
Makes 6 servings

1/2 cup extra virgin olive oil
1/8 cup tarragon vinegar
1/8 cup lemon juice
1/2 tsp. Worcestershire sauce

1 tsp. salt
fresh ground pepper to taste
dash Tabasco (optional)

Blend thoroughly with a whisk.

Calories: 166, CHO: 1g, FAT: 18g, PRO: 0g

So Simple Salad Dressing
Makes 16 servings

1 cup extra virgin olive oil
1 cup balsamic vinegar (or vinegar of choice)

Mix. Store at room temperature. Always ready to serve.

Calories: 116, CHO: 2g, FAT: 12g, PRO: 0g

Apple Flax Vinaigrette
Makes 12 servings

1/4 cup cider vinegar
2 tsp. Dijon mustard
1/2 tsp. ground coriander
1/2 tsp. cracked black pepper

1/2 cup flaxseed oil
1/4 cup extra virgin olive oil
1 cup apple cider
2 tbs. shoyu, tamari or reduced-sodium soy sauce

In a medium bowl, combine vinegar, mustard, coriander and pepper. Add oils and whisk together until well blended and emulsified. Whisk in cider and shoyu until well combined. Store in airtight container in the refrigerator up to one week.

Calories: 125.5, CHO: 1g, FAT: 13.5g, PRO: 0g

Greek Salad Dressing
Makes 16 servings (1-1/2 tbs. each)

3/4 cup extra virgin olive oil
3/4 cup high oleic safflower oil
2/3 cup garlic flavored red wine vinegar
2 tbs. honey

2 tsp. seasoned salt
1 tsp. basil
1 tsp. dry mustard
1 tsp. pepper

Mix all ingredients in a food processor or blender. Refrigerate.
This is also a great meat marinade.

Calories: 134, CHO: 2g, FAT: 14g, PRO: 0g

Summer Salsa

Makes 6 servings (1-1/2 tbs. each)

3 fresh tomatoes, chopped
1 bunch green onions
(including green tops), sliced

3 tbs. extra virgin olive oil
3 tbs. balsamic vinegar
1 tbs. minced basil

Combine all ingredients. Stir well. Cover and chill.

Calories: 95, CHO: 7g, FAT: 7g, PRO: 1g

Vegetable-Tomato Sauce

Makes 4 servings

1 medium onion, chopped
1 lb. mushrooms, sliced
1 clove garlic, minced
2 zucchini, sliced

1 red bell pepper, chopped
1–28 oz. can tomato sauce
1/4 cup chopped fresh flat-leaf parsley
1 cup kale or spinach, chopped

In large pot, combine onion, mushrooms and garlic with 1 tbs. water. Cook over high heat about 4 minutes, stirring frequently. Add zucchini, bell pepper, tomato sauce, parsley and salt and pepper to taste. Cook 1 hour, uncovered, over medium-low heat, stirring occasionally. Stir in kale or spinach. Cook just until greens wilt, 2 to 3 minutes. Serve over baked redskin potatoes.

Calories: 119, CHO: 15g, FAT: 3g, PRO: 8g

Red Pepper Dip

Makes 2 cups

2 medium red bell peppers, halved lengthwise
1 large red onion, 1/4-inch slices
2 cloves garlic, peeled
1/4 cup dry, whole grain bread crumbs

1/4 cup plain low-fat yogurt
1 tbs. red wine vinegar
2 tsp. extra virgin olive oil
1/4 cup chopped cilantro (optional)

Place pepper halves, skin sides up, on foil-lined baking sheet. Arrange onion slices and garlic around peppers. Broil 6 to 8 inches from heat source, until vegetables are blackened, about 10 minutes. Place vegetables in paper bag, seal and let stand for 15 minutes. Remove blackened skin of peppers. In food processor, combine peppers, onion and garlic and process until finely chopped. Add remaining ingredients and process until smooth. Transfer mixture to bowl. Fold in cilantro. Season with salt and pepper to taste and serve. Store in refrigerator.

Per 1 tbs. serving: Calories: 37, CHO: 5g, FAT: 1g, PRO: 2g

Soups/Chilis

Chicken Noodle Soup
Makes 8 servings

1 whole chicken (4 lbs.), cut up	1 bag frozen green beans
1 bunch celery, diced	1 bag frozen fat-free noodles
1 bag baby carrots	2 sticks cinnamon
6 small whole onions	salt and pepper to taste

Put chicken in a large stock pot with a bouquet garni of cinnamon, 1 onion, 1 carrot and celery leaves. Cover with water and boil gently for 1 hour until chicken is tender. Remove chicken and bouquet garni from broth; reserve chicken. If desired, strain broth and chill overnight to remove fat. Add remaining vegetables, except green beans, to broth and simmer gently until tender. Bone the chicken and dice or pull, then add to the heated broth and simmer until chicken is thoroughly reheated. Add green beans and noodles; heat until noodles are tender. Serve.

Calories: 380, CHO: 27g, FAT: 16g, PRO: 32g

Ostrich Soup
Makes 6 servings

1-1/2 lbs. ground ostrich	1 green pepper, chopped
1 onion, chopped	1/2 red pepper, chopped
32 oz. tomato puree	2 cups kale or spinach, chopped
32 oz. water	1 cup celery, chopped
2 cups sliced green beans	salt and pepper to taste
4 minced garlic cloves	

Brown meat in soup pot, stirring to separate meat particles and incorporate brown bits. Add onion and cook until tender. Combine remaining ingredients and simmer for 1 hour.

This is an excellent tasting, nutritious soup. Give it a try.

Calories: 336, CHO: 25g, FAT: 12g, PRO: 32g

Sweet Potato Minestrone

Makes 7 servings (1-1/2 cup each)

1/2 lb. lean ground turkey or ostrich
1 cup onion, diced
1 cup carrots, diced
3/4 cup celery, thinly sliced
2 cups peeled sweet potato, diced
2–14.5 oz. cans no-salt-added whole tomatoes, chopped, and their liquid
1–15 oz. can Great Northern beans, rinsed and drained
8 cups spinach, coarsely chopped

1 tsp. dried oregano
1/2 tsp. coarsely ground pepper
1/4 tsp. salt
3 cups water

Combine meat, onion, carrots and celery in a large sauce pan over medium-high heat; sauté 7 minutes, stirring to separate meat particles and incorporate brown bits, or until meat is browned. Add water and all remaining ingredients except spinach. Bring to a boil; cover, reduce heat and simmer for 30 minutes or until vegetables are tender. Stir in spinach; cook an additional 2 minutes.

Calories: 276, CHO: 34g, FAT: 8g, PRO: 17g

White Chili

Makes 6-8 servings

5 boneless chicken breasts, steamed and cubed
1–15 oz. jar Great Northern beans, rinsed and drained
1–12 oz. jar salsa
salt and pepper to taste

Combine all ingredients in a large saucepan. Heat thoroughly. Fast and Easy.

Calories: 292, CHO: 17g, FAT: 12g, PRO: 29g

Turkey Chili

Makes 10 servings (1-1/2 cups each)

1 lb. extra-lean ground turkey
2 onions, diced
1 tsp. minced garlic
1 cup shredded carrots
1 red pepper, chopped
1 green pepper, chopped
2–15 oz. cans black beans,
  rinsed and drained
1–15 oz. can garbanzo beans,
  rinsed and drained

1–15 oz. can kidney beans,
  rinsed and drained
1/2 tsp. red pepper flakes
1/2 tsp. cayenne pepper
1 tbs. chili powder
1 tsp. oregano
1 tbs. extra virgin olive oil
2–32 oz. bottles low-sodium V-8™ juice
1–14-oz. can stewed tomatoes
1 tbs. ground cumin

Heat oil in large pot. Add garlic, vegetables and turkey. Sauté for 5 minutes, stirring to separate meat particles. Add beans to pot. Add all spices, oil, V-8 juice and stewed tomatoes and simmer 15 minutes.

Calories: 256, CHO: 16g, FAT: 12g, PRO: 21g

Tortilla Soup
Makes 4 servings

1 tbs. extra virgin olive oil

1 large onion, chopped

1 jalapeño pepper, seeded and finely chopped

1 clove garlic, minced

1 small zucchini, sliced 1/2-inch thick

1 cup canned whole tomatoes, drained and chopped

3 cups low-sodium vegetable broth

1-1/2 cups black beans, rinsed and drained

1/2 tsp. dried oregano

2 tbs. fresh lime juice

4 tbs. shredded cheese (optional)

4 tsp. chopped cilantro (optional)

2 cups high oleic safflower-oil
yellow tortilla chips

In large saucepan, heat oil over medium-high heat. Add onion, jalapeño and garlic and cook, stirring often, until onion is slightly soft, about 4 to 5 minutes. Add zucchini, tomatoes, broth, black beans and oregano. Cook, stirring occasionally, until zucchini is almost soft, about 3 minutes. Stir in lime juice. Ladle soup into bowls and top each serving with some cheese and cilantro, if using; top with tortilla chips. Serve hot.

Calories: 276, CHO: 39g, FAT: 8g, PRO: 12g

Gazpacho
Makes 4 servings

1 small can tomato paste

2 cans water

2 small gloves garlic

1 green pepper, coarsely chopped

1 red pepper, coarsely chopped

1 yellow pepper, coarsely chopped

1 medium onion, coarsely chopped

2 fresh tomatoes or 1 can diced tomatoes, drained

1 oz. red wine vinegar

1 large cucumber

1/2 cup whole grain bread crumbs

2 tbs. extra virgin olive oil
or expeller pressed canola oil

Blend tomato paste and water. Add remaining ingredients to blender. Use "chop" button until everything is well mixed. Add bread crumbs and whip until well blended. Chill and serve.

Add spices to taste (recommended: fresh ground pepper, paprika, 1 tsp. concentrated lemon juice).

Calories: 196, CHO: 26g, FAT: 8g, PRO: 5g

Chicken Stew
Makes 4 servings

1 tbs. extra virgin olive oil
1 garlic clove, pressed
1 large onion, chopped
4 small boneless chicken breasts
4 carrots, sliced
6 small redskin potatoes, cut in small pieces

1-15 oz. can tomatoes, chopped
1 tsp. cinnamon
pinch of Cayenne pepper
1 tsp. ground cumin
2 tbs. natural chunky peanut butter
1-1/2 cups chicken broth
salt and pepper to taste

Sauté garlic and onion in olive oil. Add chicken and brown on both sides. Add the rest of the ingredients except chicken broth and stir until blended. Then add the broth and seasonings to taste. Cook over medium-low heat until sauce thickens, about 50 minutes.

Calories: 406, CHO: 30g, FAT: 18g, PRO: 31g

Cream of Mushroom Soup with Chicken
Makes 4 servings

1 tbs. extra virgin olive oil
1 lb. fresh mushrooms, sliced
1/2 cup chopped onion
1/4 cup + 3/4 cup evaporated skim milk

16 oz. defatted chicken broth
2 tbs. cornstarch
2 boneless chicken breasts,
    steamed or sautéed, cubed

Coat saucepan with extra virgin olive oil. Sauté mushrooms and onion until tender. Transfer half of vegetables to blender, add broth and process until smooth. In small bowl, stir cornstarch and 1/4 cup milk until smooth. Combine mushroom and cornstarch mixtures. Add remaining milk, vegetables and chicken. Cook and stir over medium heat until soup thickens.

Calories: 292, CHO: 26g, FAT: 12g, PRO: 20g

Entrees

Lasagna
Makes 9 servings

2 tbs. extra virgin olive oil
5 cups onion, thinly sliced
3 garlic cloves, thinly sliced
1 cup green bell pepper, thinly sliced
2 cups red bell pepper, thinly sliced
1 cup yellow bell pepper, thinly sliced
8–3.5 oz. links sweet Italian sausage,
 cooked and drained

1/2 cup shredded part-skim
 Mozzarella cheese
2-1/4 cups prepared fat-free tomato basil
 pasta sauce (Millina's Finest™)
6–7 x 3 1/2 inch no-boil lasagna noodles (Vigo™)
1/2 cup grated fresh Parmesan cheese
6 oz. block-style fat-free cream cheese,
 cut into bite-size pieces

Preheat oven to 350°. Mix all ingredients except noodles and cheeses in bowl.
In large pan, layer noodles, sauce mixture and cheeses, ending with cheese layer.
Bake 45 minutes. Let stand 5–10 minutes before slicing.

Calories: 379.5, CHO: 33g, FAT: 15.5g, PRO: 27g

Chicken Quesadillas
Makes 4 servings

1 tbs. extra virgin olive oil
2 boneless chicken breasts
1 large red or green pepper, chopped
1 medium onion, chopped

1 cup mild salsa
1/2 cup Cheddar-Veggie Shreds™
1 large tomato, diced
2 large whole wheat lavash

Coat large, non-stick frying pan with half of oil. Cut chicken into small chunks
and sauté until cooked through. Remove chicken and sauté peppers and onion until
tender. Set aside. Coat pan again with oil. Place 1 lavash in pan. Scatter half of chicken,
vegetables, cheese and salsa over one half of the lavash. Fold other half of lavash over
chicken mixture. Heat on medium until bottom is lightly browned. Turn over and heat
until cheese is melted. Repeat with second lavash. Cut into triangles.

Calories: 385, CHO: 51g, FAT: 9g, PRO: 25g

Chicken Pasta
Makes 3 servings

3 boneless, skinless chicken breasts
2 egg whites (free-range eggs), lightly beaten
pinch seasoning salt
pinch Cayenne pepper
1/2 cup whole grain breadcrumbs

1 tbs. expeller pressed canola oil
3/4 cup tomato sauce (optional)
fat-free Parmesan cheese (optional)
3 cups whole grain pasta, cooked

Brush skinless, boneless chicken breasts with two egg whites, and lightly roll in breadcrumbs. Season with seasoning salt, and Cayenne pepper. Heat oil in a skillet, and cook chicken until golden brown (approximately 5 minutes per side). Top each portion with 1/4 cup of your favorite tomato sauce, if using, and sprinkle with fat-free Parmesan cheese. Serve over 1 cup whole grain pasta.

Calories: 401, CHO: 55.5g, FAT: 7g, PRO: 29g

Sloppy Joes
Makes 7 or 8 servings

1 lb. ground turkey or tempeh
1 cup onion, chopped
1/2 cup celery, chopped
2 tbs. extra virgin olive oil or canola oil
1–15 oz. can tomato sauce
2 tbs. rolled oats
1 tsp. Worcestershire sauce

1/2 tsp. chili powder
dash hot pepper sauce
1/2 cup water
1 tsp. salt
1/8 tsp. pepper
whole grain rolls or bread (1 per
  serving)

In skillet, cook turkey or tempeh, onion and celery in oil until browned. Stir in tomato sauce, oats, Worcestershire sauce, chili powder, hot pepper sauce, water, salt and pepper. Simmer, uncovered, about 30 minutes. Spoon about 1/2 cup of mixture onto each roll or slice of bread.

Calories: 124.5, CHO: 7g, FAT: 4.5g, PRO: 14g [without roll or bread]

Vegetarian BBQ
Makes 6 servings

10-1/2 oz. package frozen bite-size
  soy "meat", thawed
1 clove garlic, minced
1 tbs. tomato paste
1 medium onion, finely chopped

1 cup barbecue sauce
1 tbs. brown mustard
1 tsp. maple syrup
1 tbs. extra virgin olive oil
6 whole grain rolls or hamburger buns

Chop soy meat into 1/2-inch pieces. Place in bowl along with all ingredients except for the olive oil and the rolls. Set aside and let stand for 10 minutes so flavors meld. Grill whole grain rolls or buns for 2-4 minutes. In medium skillet, heat oil over medium-high heat. Add soy meat and marinade. Reduce heat and simmer, stirring occasionally, for about 10 minutes (until sauce thickens). Spoon BBQ mixture over rolls or buns and serve. Can be frozen in single servings, then reheated in the microwave for instant meals!

Calories: 291, CHO: 32g, FAT: 3g, PRO: 34g

Turkey Burgers or Meatloaf
Makes 8 servings

1-1/2 lbs. lean ground turkey
1–10 oz. package frozen chopped spinach
  (thawed and drained) OR 1/2 cup green
  or red bell pepper, finely chopped
2 egg whites (free-range eggs)
1-1/2 tsp. Italian seasoning

1 cup rolled oats
1/2 cup onion, chopped
1/2 cup carrots, shredded
1 small apple, shredded
1/3 cup skim milk
1/2 tsp. salt
1/4 tsp. pepper

Preheat oven to 350°. Combine all ingredients in large bowl; mix thoroughly.
Shape into loaf in 13 x 9 baking pan. Bake 45 to 50 minutes or until done. Let stand
5 minutes before slicing. For burgers, form into patties and broil, bake or grill as desired.

Calories: 199, CHO: 13g, FAT: 7g, PRO: 21g

Chicken and Vegetable Pizza
Makes 8 servings

2 chicken breasts, chunked
1 tbs. expeller pressed canola oil or
  extra virgin olive oil
1 small onion, sliced
1/2 green bell pepper, sliced
1/2 red bell pepper, sliced

1/3 cup mango, pineapple, or peach chutney
1-8 oz. can pineapple tidbits, drained
1 cup reduced-fat Mozzarella cheese, shredded
1–12 in. ready-made pizza crust

Preheat oven to 450°. Sauté chicken, onion and peppers in oil until chicken is no longer pink. Spread chutney evenly on ready-made pizza crust. Spread chicken mixture and pineapple tidbits over chutney. Sprinkle Mozzarella cheese on top. Bake for 10 to 12 minutes and cut into 8 slices.

Calories: 217.5, CHO: 28g, FAT: 5.5g, PRO: 14g

Mexican Pizza
Makes 2 servings

1 tbs. extra virgin olive oil
2 flour tortillas (8-inch, non-hydrogenated)
1/2 cup salsa, drained
1/4 cup canned red kidney beans, rinsed and drained
1/4 cup canned black beans, rinsed and drained

1 tbs. chopped fresh cilantro
1/3 cup reduced-fat hot pepper
   Monterey Jack cheese, shredded

Preheat oven to 375°. Coat a baking sheet lightly with extra virgin olive oil. Place the tortillas on the baking sheet. Coat each tortilla with oil. Spoon half the salsa onto each tortilla. Sprinkle with beans, cheese and cilantro. Bake 10 to 15 minutes or until cheese is melted.

Calories: 284, CHO: 48g, FAT: 0g, PRO: 23g

Chicken Stir-Fry
Makes 4 servings

8 chicken breast tenders
1 tbs. extra virgin olive oil or
   expeller pressed canola oil, divided
1 cup carrots, sliced
1 cup mushrooms, sliced

1 tbs. soy sauce
2 cups cabbage, shredded
1 cup bean sprouts
3 tbs. natural peanut butter

Steam, or sauté chicken using 1/2 tbs. oil; cut into bite-size pieces and set aside. Stir-fry vegetables in oil to desired tenderness. Combine chicken with vegetables. Stir in natural peanut butter and soy sauce.

Calories: 236, CHO: 10g, FAT: 8g, PRO: 31g

Yogurt Chicken
Makes 7 servings

2 lbs. skinless chicken thighs (bone-in)
2 tbs. lemon or lime juice
1 tbs. extra virgin olive oil or
   expeller pressed canola oil
1 cup plain low-fat yogurt
3 tbs. canola oil mayonnaise
   (low-fat if desired)

1 tbs. Dijon style mustard
1 tbs. Worcestershire sauce
1/3 tsp. dried thyme or 2 tsp. fresh
1/4 cup green onion (including green
   tops), sliced
1/4 tsp. Cayenne pepper, or to taste
1/4 cup fresh Parmesan cheese, grated

Preheat oven to 350°. Blend together lemon and oil and coat chicken thighs. Place in a shallow baking dish and bake, uncovered, for approximately 50 minutes. Remove from oven and drain off all accumulated juices. Blend remaining ingredients except Parmesan and spread over chicken. Sprinkle Parmesan on top. Return to oven and broil until cheese has melted and begins to brown.

Calories: 226, CHO: 5g, FAT: 10g, PRO: 29g

Baked Chicken and Vegetables
Makes 4 servings

4 carrots, sliced thick
2 large potatoes, sliced thick
2 sweet potatoes, sliced thick
4 skinless, boneless chicken breasts

2 yellow onions, sliced thin
1-1/2 cups water
1/8 cup slivered almonds

Preheat oven to 350°. Place carrots and potato slices in a casserole dish and place chicken breasts on top. Cover with onion slices. Pour water over ingredients; cover casserole dish. Bake for 1-1/2 hours, until tender. Sprinkle slivered almonds on top and serve.

Calories: 304, CHO: 36g, FAT: 4g, PRO: 31g

No-Fry Chicken
Makes 4 servings

4 skinless, boneless chicken breasts
3/4 cup plain non-fat yogurt
1 tbs. spicy mustard

1/2 cup dry bread crumbs
1/2 cup unbleached flour
1 tbs. extra virgin olive oil

Preheat oven to 400°. Cool chicken in ice water; remove and pat dry with paper towel. Combine yogurt and mustard in small bowl. Combine bread crumbs and flour in small bowl. Dip chicken in yogurt mixture then roll in bread crumb mixture. Place on oiled baking sheet. Bake 30 to 40 minutes or until cooked through, turning halfway through to brown bottom.

Calories: 269.5, CHO: 21g, FAT: 7.5g, PRO: 29.5g

Orange Chicken and Rice
Makes 4 servings

1 lb. skinless, boneless chicken thighs,
  cut into 2-inch pieces
1–2 tbs. expeller pressed canola oil
  or extra virgin olive oil
1 medium onion, coarsely chopped
1-1/2 cups orange juice
1–14 oz. can chicken broth
2 cloves garlic, minced or pressed in a garlic press

1/3 tsp. curry
dash of cinnamon
3 tbs. raisins (optional)
1/2 cup rice, whole grain
salt and pepper to taste

Sauté chicken and onion in oil until brown. Add the broth, orange juice, garlic and seasonings. Cover and cook over low heat for 45 minutes. Add raisins and rice to the same pot, lower the heat and simmer 25 minutes or until rice is done (check package for directions). Add more water or broth if sauce is too thick. Salt and pepper to taste.

Calories: 253, CHO: 18g, FAT: 9g, PRO: 25g

Confetti Wrap

Makes 2 servings

2 tbs. canola light mayonnaise
1/2 tsp. mustard
1–6 oz. can boneless, water-packed, skinless
salmon or albacore tuna, drained

1/2 package broccoli slaw mix
1/2 small onion, diced
2 fat-free flour tortillas

Blend mayonnaise and mustard. Add remaining ingredients and mix well. Enjoy as a salad or wrap in the tortillas. For variety, add sliced grapes or a few broken walnuts.

Calories: 228.5, CHO: 21g, FAT: 4.5g, PRO: 26g

Salmon or Tuna Patties

Makes 4 or 5 servings

1–16 oz. can salmon or tuna
1/2 cup onion, chopped
4 egg whites (free-range eggs)
1/3 cup + 1/3 cup bread crumbs, cracker crumbs or rolled oats

2 tbs. soy or skim milk
2 tbs. extra virgin olive oil or canola oil

Drain salmon or tuna, discard bones and skin; flake meat. Combine with onion, 1/3 cup bread crumbs, egg whites and milk; mix well. Shape into 4 or 5 patties; coat with remaining bread crumbs. Cook patties over medium heat in oil about 3 minutes or until browned. Carefully turn; brown other side, about 3 minutes more.

Calories: 274, CHO: 15.5g, FAT: 12g, PRO: 26g

Grilled Salmon and Vegetables

Makes 3–4 servings

1-1/2 lbs. salmon fillets
1 eggplant, sliced 1/2-inch thick

4 or 5 large Portobello mushrooms, sliced
1 red bell pepper, sliced

Marinade

1/3 cup extra virgin olive oil
1/4 cup lemon or lime juice
1 to 3 cloves garlic, minced

1/2 tsp. paprika
1/2 tsp. cumin

Mix marinade ingredients in large bowl. Marinate salmon and vegetables in bowl for 1 hour. Remove fish and vegetables from marinade; discard marinade. Grill or broil salmon and vegetables.

Calories: 398, CHO: 14g, FAT: 22g, PRO: 36g [with marinade]

Salmon Teriyaki

Makes 4 servings

2 lbs. salmon fillets
8 fresh green onions (including green
  tops), chopped
12 slices fresh ginger

1/2 cup light teriyaki sauce
  or Bragg's Liquid Aminos
2 or 2-2/3 cups cooked brown rice or
  8 small cooked redskin potatoes

Preheat oven to 425°. Place salmon in shallow baking dish, skin side down. Sprinkle onions over salmon and scatter ginger slices. Pour teriyaki or Bragg's over the salmon. Cover tightly with foil. Bake 20 minutes or until fish flakes. Serve with 1/2–2/3 cup cooked brown rice or 2 small redskin potatoes.

Calories: 326.5, CHO: 9g, FAT: 14.5g, PRO: 40g

Paprika-Cumin Salmon Fillets

Makes 4–6 servings

2 lbs. skinned salmon fillets, cut into 4 pieces
1 tsp. ground cumin
1/2 tsp. salt

1 tsp. paprika
1/2 tsp. ground pepper
1/2 tsp. extra virgin olive oil

Combine spices and sprinkle on both sides of fish. Coat a non-stick skillet with oil and add fish. Cook on medium heat 6 minutes on each side or until fish flakes easily.

Calories: 294, CHO: 2g, FAT: 14g, PRO: 40g

Red Snapper

Makes 4 servings

1-1/2 lbs. red snapper
garlic powder, to taste
black pepper, to taste
Cajun spice, to taste

onion powder, to taste
Cayenne pepper, to taste
seasoning salt, to taste
lemon juice, to taste

Preheat oven to 400°. Season both sides of the red snapper with the spices. Bake for about 12 minutes, until fish flakes and juices are clear. Squeeze lemon juice over the snapper. Serve with 1/2-2/3 cup cooked brown rice or 2 small redskin potatoes with a sprinkle of extra virgin olive oil.

Calories: 202, CHO: 1g, FAT: 6g, PRO: 36g [fish only]

Barbecued Pork or Beef Tenderloin
Makes 4 servings

1-1/2 lbs. pork or beef tenderloin	barbecue sauce
4 tbs. natural applesauce	dash cinnamon

Grill tenderloin while brushing it with barbecue sauce until the meat is no longer pink (approximately 5 minutes each side). Thinly slice the meat; divide into 4 portions and top each with natural applesauce sprinkled with cinnamon. Serve over 1/2–2/3 cup cooked brown rice.

Calories: 338, CHO: 34g, FAT: 6g, PRO: 37g

Pork Loin Chops and Peppers
Makes 6 servings

6 pork loin chops	1/4 cup water
salt and pepper, to taste	8 oz. mushrooms, sliced
1/4 tsp. rosemary	1 green bell pepper,
2 tbs. expeller pressed canola oil	sliced into long thin strips
or extra virgin olive oil	1 red bell pepper,
1 onion, sliced	sliced into long thin strips

Cream Sauce

2 tbs. expeller pressed canola oil	1/4 cup flour
or extra virgin olive oil	2 cups soy or skim milk

Season chops with salt, pepper and rosemary; brown in oil over medium heat. Lower temperature to simmer and add onion and water. Cover and cook slowly for 20 minutes.

Prepare cream sauce by heating oil in saucepan; add flour and combine. Cook for 5 minutes, stirring constantly, to eliminate the flour taste. Add milk and stir until thickened. Add mushrooms, peppers and cream sauce to chops. Cover and simmer 5 to 10 minutes more.

Calories: 311.6, CHO: 12.5g, FAT: 16g, PRO: 29.4g

Baked Eggplant
Makes 6 servings

1 lb. lean ground turkey	1/2 tsp. cinnamon
2 medium onions, chopped	3 large eggplants, peeled and
1/2 tsp. salt	cut into 1/2 inch slices
1/2 tsp. pepper	1-15 oz. can tomato puree
1/2 tsp. ground allspice	3 cups cooked whole grain rice

Brown turkey in nonstick pan, stirring to separate meat particles. Add onion and seasonings. Sauté or broil eggplant till tender. Layer eggplant and turkey mixture in a 13 x 9 inch pan. Pour tomato puree over all. Bake at 375° for 20-25 minutes or until bubbly. Serve over 1/2 cup servings of rice.

Calories: 210, CHO: 27g, FAT: 2g, PRO: 21g

Desserts

Pumpkin Pie
Makes 8 servings

4 egg whites (free-range eggs)
1/4 cup sugar or Stevia Plus equivalent

1–12 oz. can evaporated skim milk
1–15 oz. can solid pack pumpkin

Preheat oven to 425°. Beat egg whites and sugar until dissolved. Add remaining ingredients and mix. Pour into 9-inch pie pan sprayed with nonstick spray. (That's right, no crust.) As an alternative, use Low-Fat Graham cracker crust (recipe below). Bake 45-60 minutes, until knife inserted in center comes out clean.

Calories: 113, CHO: 15g, FAT: 1g, PRO: 11g [without crust]

Low-Fat Graham Cracker Crust

1-1/4 cups graham cracker crumbs (Barbara's Bakery® Organic Go Go Grahams)
1/3 cup baby applesauce

Combine ingredients and press into a 9-inch pie pan sprayed with nonstick spray.

This crust will add more carbohydrates but is a better alternative to pastry crust or Graham cracker crust made with butter.

Calories: 91, CHO: 16.75g, FAT: 2g, PRO: 1.5g

Pumpkin Cookies
Makes about 36 cookies

1 cup packed light brown sugar
1/3 cup high oleic sunflower oil
1 cup canned solid pack pumpkin
1 tsp. vanilla extract
1-1/2 cups unbleached all-purpose flour
1/2 tsp. aluminum-free baking powder

1/2 tsp. baking soda
1 tsp. ground cinnamon
1/2 tsp. ground allspice
1/2 tsp. salt
1/2 cup chopped dates
1/2 cup hulled pumpkin seeds, coarsely chopped

Preheat oven to 375°. In a large bowl, combine sugar and oil. Beat with electric mixer on medium speed until well blended. Blend in pumpkin and vanilla until well blended, scraping down sides of bowl as needed. On low speed, beat in all remaining ingredients except for the dates and pumpkin seeds. Stir in pumpkin seeds and dates. Drop batter by tablespoonfuls, 2 inches apart, onto oiled cookie sheet. Using fork, press cookies to flatten slightly. Bake until lightly browned, about 15 minutes. Transfer cookies to wire rack to cool.

Calories: 89, CHO: 10g, FAT: 5g, PRO: 2g

Apple Crisp
Makes 8–10 servings

5 pounds of sliced, peeled apples
2 tsp. cinnamon
2 cups rolled oats
1 cup flour
1/4 cup packed brown sugar

1/4 tsp. salt
1 tsp. baking powder
2 free-range eggs, lightly beaten
1/2 cup Earth Balance butter spread,
   melted, or expeller pressed canola oil

Preheat oven to 350°. Toss apples with cinnamon and arrange in bottom of a 13 x 9 inch pan. Mix dry ingredients. Lightly work in eggs until mixture is crumbly. Sprinkle mixture on top of apples. Pour melted butter spread or oil evenly over the top. Bake 45 minutes.

Calories: 200, CHO: 28g, FAT: 8g, PRO: 4g

Chocolate Protein Brownies
Makes 16 servings

1/2 cup natural soy protein powder
1/2 cup sugar
5 tbs. unsweetened cocoa powder
3/4 cup flour
1/4 tsp. salt
1/4 tsp. cinnamon
3/4 tsp. baking soda

3/4 cup warm water
1 tsp. vanilla
2 tbs. expeller pressed canola oil
2 tsp. vinegar
1 egg white (free-range egg)
2 tbs. chopped walnuts (optional)

Preheat oven to 350°. Measure dry ingredients into bowl and mix well. Add warm water, vanilla, oil, vinegar and egg white. Stir until combined. Spread batter into an 8 x 8 nonstick baking pan and sprinkle with nuts. Bake 18–20 minutes.

Calories: 95, CHO: 13g, FAT: 3g, PRO: 4g

Chocolate Pie
Makes 8 servings

1 cup soy or skim milk
2 cups canned evaporated skim milk
1-1/2 cup sugar or Stevia Plus equivalent
1/3 cup cornstarch
1/2 tsp. salt

1/2 cup unsweetened cocoa powder
4 free-range eggs
1 tsp. vanilla
1 9-inch chocolate crumb pie crust
   (recipe follows)

Combine milks, sugar, cornstarch and salt in medium saucepan and whisk. Bring to near boil and whisk in cocoa. Reduce heat and simmer for 15 minutes, whisking frequently. In medium bowl, beat eggs and very slowly add 1 cup of the cocoa mixture. Return egg and cocoa mixture to the saucepan. Increase heat, bring to a boil and cook, stirring constantly, for 1 minute. Remove from heat and stir in vanilla. Pour chocolate mixture into chocolate crumb crust and cover with a sheet of waxed paper. Refrigerate 4 hours. Serve chilled.

Calories: 267, CHO: 50g, FAT: 3g, PRO: 10g [with sugar]
Calories: 183, CHO: 29g, FAT: 3g, PRO: 10g [with Stevia Plus]

Chocolate-Crumb Pie Crust

Makes one 9-inch crust

3 tbs. Earth Balance butter spread
1 oz. bittersweet chocolate, chopped
30 all-natural chocolate sandwich cookies (remove cream from cookie center)

Spray 9-inch glass pie pan with non-stick cooking spray. In small saucepan, combine butter spread and chocolate and cook over low heat until melted, stirring frequently. Finely grind cookies in food processor. Add chocolate mixture and process again until crumbs are just moistened. Press crumb mixture along bottom and sides of pie pan. Freeze for at least 30 minutes before filling.

Calories: 244, CHO: 31g, FAT: 12g, PRO: 3g

Carrot Cake

Makes 8 servings

2 tbs. expeller pressed canola oil
   or 2 free-range eggs
1 cup sugar or Stevia Plus equivalent
1 tbs. cinnamon
1-1/3 cup white or whole-wheat pastry
   flour, unsifted

1/2 cup flaxmeal or chopped walnuts
1 tsp. baking soda
1/2 tsp. salt
1-1/2 cups carrots, grated
1/2 cup raisins
1 tsp. orange peel, grated

Preheat oven to 350°. Beat oil or eggs and sugar with a mixer (or by hand) until creamy. Mix dry ingredients in a separate bowl and add to the egg mixture. Beat for an additional minute. Add remaining ingredients and stir until combined. Spoon batter into a lightly oiled, 8 x 8 inch baking pan and bake 30 to 40 minutes or until done. Cake is done when you touch it lightly in the center and it springs back.

This cake is tasty and most healthful without frostings or toppings.

Calories: 309, CHO: 40g, FAT: 13g, PRO: 8g [with sugar]
Calories: 253, CHO: 26g, FAT: 13g, PRO: 8g [with Stevia Plus]

Hazelnut Fudge Cake

Makes 8 servings

1 cup pitted prunes, chopped
1/3 cup apple juice
5 free-range eggs
2 tsp. vanilla
1-1/2 cup soy or skim milk

1-1/4 cups unsweetened cocoa powder
1 cup sugar or Stevia Plus equivalent
2 cups all-purpose flour
2 tsp. aluminum-free baking powder
1/2 cup ground hazelnuts

Preheat oven to 350°. Coat 9-inch springform pan with non-stick cooking spray. In a small saucepan, combine prunes and apple juice. Bring to a boil, reduce heat and simmer, uncovered, 5–7 minutes, or until prunes are soft. Transfer to a food processor and puree to a paste. In large bowl, combine eggs, vanilla and milk. Beat well. Beat in pureed prunes. In medium bowl, combine cocoa, sugar, flour and baking powder. Add cocoa mixture to prune mixture and stir just until combined. Mix in hazelnuts. Pour batter into a springform pan and bake 45 minutes, or until a knife inserted in center comes out with moist crumbs attached. Let cool before cutting.

Calories: 339, CHO: 52g, FAT: 11g, PRO: 8g

Cookies That "Rock"

Makes 48 cookies

1 cup whole wheat flour
1 cup rolled oats
3/4 cup flaxmeal
1/4 cup whole flaxseeds
1 tsp. baking soda
1 tsp. salt
1 cup soy protein powder

1 cup packed brown sugar
  or Stevia Plus equivalent
6 egg whites (free-range eggs)
1/2 cup natural applesauce
1 tbs. expeller pressed canola oil
1 tbs. vanilla
1 cup organic chocolate chips
3/4 cup chopped walnuts

Preheat oven to 350°. Combine dry ingredients, except chocolate chips and nuts, and mix well. Add egg whites, applesauce, oil and vanilla. Beat with electric mixer until combined. Stir in chocolate chips and nuts. Drop 1 tablespoon of dough onto oiled cookie sheet for each cookie, flattening slightly. Bake 12–14 minutes. Remove from cookie sheet and cool.

Calories: 96, CHO: 11g, FAT: 4g, PRO: 4g [per cookie]

Chapter 24

Daily Logs

Use the following logs as tools to develop and reinforce your new healthy nutrition and exercise patterns. Start slowly and make small changes.

EXERCISE LOG
WEEK OF ____ / ____ / ____

	Warm-Up Stretching	Cardiovascular Exercise	Strength Training	Balance / Flexibility	Daily Physical Activity	Comments
MON						
TUE						
WED						
THU						
FRI						
SAT						
SUN						

DAILY FOOD LOG   Day: _____   Date: _____

Meal	Description	Target
Breakfast Time:		
Snack 1 Time:		
Lunch Time:		
Snack 2 Time:		
Dinner Time:		
Snack 3 Time:		

Water (8oz)	☐ ☐ ☐ ☐ ☐ ☐ ☐ ☐ ☐ ☐		
Sleep (hours)	4 ☐ 5 ☐ 6 ☐ 7 ☐ 8 ☐ 9 ☐ 10 ☐		
Activity / Exercise	☐ Cardio ☐ Strength ☐ Flexibility ☐ Other		
Comments			

Food Target

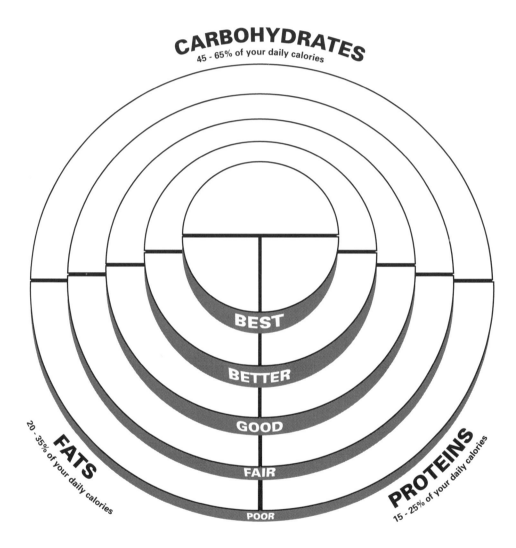

Meal Patterning Food Log

DAILY FOOD LOG   Day: _____   Date:_____

Meal	Description	Target
Breakfast Time: _____		CARBOHYDRATES / FATS / PROTEINS
Snack 1 Time: _____		CARBOHYDRATES / FATS / PROTEINS
Lunch Time: _____		CARBOHYDRATES / FATS / PROTEINS
Snack 2 Time: _____		CARBOHYDRATES / FATS / PROTEINS
Dinner Time: _____		CARBOHYDRATES / FATS / PROTEINS
Snack 3 Time: _____		CARBOHYDRATES / FATS / PROTEINS

Water (8oz)	☐ ☐ ☐ ☐ ☐ ☐ ☐ ☐ ☐ ☐
Sleep (hours)	4 ☐ 5 ☐ 6 ☐ 7 ☐ 8 ☐ 9 ☐ 10 ☐
Activity / Exercise	☐ Cardio ☐ Strength ☐ Flexibility ☐ Other
Comments	

Meal Patterning Exercise Log

EXERCISE LOG

WEEK OF ___/___/___

	Warm-Up Stretching	Cardiovascular Exercise	Strength Training	Balance / Flexibility	Daily Physical Activity	Comments
MON						
TUE						
WED						
THU						
FRI						
SAT						
SUN						

Bibliography

"Aspartame: It isn't as sweet as you think." "Aspartame/NutraSweet Dangers in Pregnancy." Aspartame (NutraSweet) Toxicity Info Center.

"Nutrition and Your Health: Dietary Guidelines for Americans." U.S. Department of Agriculture, 2000: Washington, D.C.

betternutrition.com, "The Joy of Soy." Jan. 2003.

"The New Glucose Revolution"

"Impotence: NIH Consensus Conference." *Journal of the American Medical Association*, 1993. 270: 83-90.

"Fat intake continues to drop; veggies, fruits still low in US diet." *Research News*. 1996.

"Economic Consequences of Diabetes Mellitus in the U.S. in 1997." 1997. American Dietetics Association.

"Mediterranean Diet, Traditional Risk Factors, and the Rate of Cardiovascular Complications after Myocardial Infarction: Final Report of Lion Diet Heart Study." *Circulation*, 1999. 1999: 779-85.

"Turn Back the Clock with Nature's Fountain of Youth." *Health Science Institute*. 2000. 1-5.

"Why You Need to Protect Your Liver." *Consumer Reports on Health*. 2001. 6-9.

"Bottled Water." *Detroit Free Press*. 2002: Detroit, MI.

"Tomorrow's Medicine Today." *Health and Healing*, Dec 1994. 4(12): 1-3.

"U.S. Surgeon General Launches Campaign to Combat Obesity." *Club Business International*. March 2002. 17.

"All Fish Are Not Created Equal." *Prevention*. Nov 2000.

CA. A Cancer Journal for Clinicians. 2001. 51(3): 182-187.

"The Newest Childhood Disease: Type 2 Diabetes," *Prevention*. Nov 2001.

"Flaxseed Facts." *Prevention*. Oct 2001. 68.

"Taking Charge of Diabetes." *Consumer Reports*. Oct 2001. 34-37.

Abraham, G.E., "The Calcium Controversy." *Journal of Applied Nutrition*, 1982. 34: 69.

Abraham, G.E. and H. Grewal, "A Total Dietary Program Emphasizing Magnesium Instead of Calcium: Effect on the Mineral Density of Calcaneous Bone in Post Menopausal Women on Hormonal Therapy." *Journal of Reproductive Medicine*, 1990. 35: 503.

Alexander, J.L., "The Role of Resistance Exercise in Weight Loss." *Strength and Conditioning Journal*, 2002: 65-70.

Anderson, A.J.C., *Refining of Oils and Fats*. ed. K.V. Williams. 1962, Elmsford: Pergamon Press.

Anderson, J.W., et. al., "Dietary Fiber and Diabetes: A Comprehensive Review And Practical Application." *Journal of the American Dietetic Association*, 1987. 1987(9): 1189-1197.

Anggard, E., *Nitric Oxide: Mediator, Murderer, and Medicine*. Lancet, 1994. 343: 1199-1207.

Atkins, R.C., *Dr. Atkin's Diet Revolution*. 1972, New York: Bantam Books.

Austad, S.N., *Why We Age*. 1997, New York: John Wiley & Sons.

Balch, J.F. and P.A. Balch, *Prescription for Nutritional Healing*. 2 ed. 1997, Garden City: Avery Publishing Group.

Baldwin, B.E., "Soy on Trial." *Journal of Health & Healing*. 24(2): 14-16.

Batmanghelidj, F., M.D., *Your Body's Many Cries For Water.* 2 ed. 1997, Vienna: Global Health Solutions Inc.

Belury, M.A. and J.P. Vanden Heuval, "Protection Against Cancer and Heart Disease by the Dietary Fatty Acid, Conjugated Linoleic Acid: Potential Mechanisms of Action." *Nutrition and Disease Update Journal*, 1997. 1(2): 53-58.

Berdanier, C.D., "Diabetes Mellitus: Is There a Connection with Infant-feeding Practices?" *Nutrition Today*. Sep/Oct 2001. 241-248.

Beutler, J., "High in Lignan Flax Oil." *Health Perspectives.* 1997. 1-2.

Brand-Miller, J., et. al. *The New Glucose Revolution.* 2003. Marlowe & Co.

Booth, S., "Flaxseed Improves Blood Glucose Levels." *Journal of Human Nutrition & Dietetics*, 2000. 13: 363-371.

Buchanan, H.M., and et. al., "Is Diet Important to Rheumatoid Arthritis?" *British Journal of Rheumatology*, 1991. 30(2): 125-34.

Budwig, J., Dr., *The Oil Protein Diet Cookbook.* 1994, Vancouver: Apple Publishing Company, Ltd.

Cabot, S., *The Liver Cleansing Diet.* 1996, Scottsdale: SCB International.

Carey, B., *Risks of Ephedra Usage in Spotlight*, ACE Certified News: Los Angeles. 11-12.

Caroll, K.K., "Review of Clinical Studies on Cholesterol-Lowering Response to Soy Protein." *Journal of the American Dietetic Association*, 1991. 1991: 820-827.

Carper, J., "The Little Antioxidant with Big Benefits." *USA Weekend.* 2002. 6.

Cherniske, S., *Caffeine Blues.* 1998, New York: Warner Books.

Clarkson, P.M., "Effects of Exercise on Chromium Levels. Is Supplementation Required?" *Sports Medicine*, 1997. 23(6): 341-9.

Cohen, L.A., "Nutrition and Cancer Prevention: Differing Perspectives on the Best Research to Achieve It." *Nutrition Today*. Mar/Apr 2001. 78-79.

Colgan, M., Dr., *The New Nutrition: Medicine for the Millennium*. 1994, Vancouver: Apple Publishing.

Colgan, M., Dr., *Hormonal Health*. 1 ed. 1996, Vancouver: Apple Publishing.

Colquhoun, I. and S. Bunday, "A Lack of Essential Fatty Acids as a Possible Cause of Hyperactivity in Children." *Medical Hypotheses*. 1981. 7: 673.

Coulombe, R.A. and R.P. Sharma, "Neurobiochemical Alterations Induced by the Artificial Sweetener Aspartame." *Toxicology and Applied Pharmacology*, 1986. 83: 79-85.

Coyle, J.T. and et. al., "Alzheimer's Disease: A Disorder of Cortical Cholinergic Innervation." *Science*, 1983. 219: 1184-1190.

Craig, B.W. and et. al., "Effects of Progressive Resistance Training on Growth Hormone and Testosterone Levels in Young and Elderly Men." *Mechanisms of Aging and Development*, 1989. 49: 159-169.

Cumming, D.C., *Hormones and Athletic Performance*. 3 ed, ed. P. Felig, J.D. Baxter, and L.A. Frohman. 1995, New York: McGraw-Hill.

Cunnane, S.C. and et. al., "Nutritional Attributes of Traditional Flaxseed in Healthy Young Adults." *American Journal of Clinical Nutrition*, 1995.61(1): 62-68.

Curtis, D., "Pump Up Your Protein Powder?" *Muscle & Fitness*. 1991. 75.

Dawson, T.M. and V.L. Dawson, "Nitric Oxide: Actions and Pathological Roles." *The Neuroscientist*, 1994. 1: 920.

Dyer, R., "Helping Your Clients Lose Weight." *Personal Fitness Professional*. 2002. 38-40.

Eaton, S.B., M. Shosstak, and M. Konner, *The Paleolithic Prescription*. 1988, New York: Harper & Row.

Enig, M., *Trans Fatty Acids in the Food Supply: A Comprehensive Report Covering 60 Years of Research*. 1993, Silver Spring: Enig Associates.

Epel, E.S. and et. al., "Stress-Induced Cortisol, Mood, and Fat Distribution." *Men. Obesity Research*, 1999. 7(1): 9-15.

Epel, E.S. and et. al., "Stress and Body Shape: Stress-Induced Cortisol Secretion is Consistently Greater Among Women with Central Fat." *Psychosomatic Medicine*, 2000. 62(5).

Erasmus, U., *Fats that Heal Fats that Kill*. 1993, Burmby: Alive Books.

Erin, D., "The Missing Nutritional Link That Cured My Ten Years of Schizophrenia" *Alternative Medicine Digest*, 1995. 7: 10-13.

Eschwege, E., et. al., "Coronary Heart Disease Mortality in Relation with Diabetes, Blood Glucose, and Plasma Insulin Levels." *Hormone and Metabolic Research Supplement*, 1985. 15: 41-46.

Fanaian, M., et. al., "The Effect of Modified Fat Diet on Insulin Resistance and Metabolic Parameters in Type II Diabetes." *Diabetologia*, 1996. 39: A7.

Felig, P., J.D. Baxter, and L.A. Frohman, *Endocrinology and Metabolism*. 1995, New York: McGraw-Hill.

Feskanich, D. and et. al., "Protein Consumption and Bone Fractures in Women." *American Journal of Epidemiology*, 1996. 143: 472-79.

Feskanich, D. and et. al., "Milk, Dietary Calcium, and Bone Fractures in Women: A 12-year Prospective Study." *American Journal of Public Health*, 1997. 87: 992-97.

Foster-Powell, K., et. al. "International table of glycemic index and glycemic load Values." *American Journal of Clinical Nutrition.* 2002. 76: 5-56.

Galli, C. and A.P. Simopoulos, eds., *Dietary W-3 and W-6 Fatty Acids: Biological Effects and Nutritional Essentiality.* 1989, New York: Plenum Publishing.

Gittleman, A.L., *The 40/30/30 Phenomenon.* 1997, New Canaan: Keats Publishing.

Gittleman, A.L., *Eat Fat, Lose Weight.* 1999, Lincolnwood: Keats Publishing.

Gittleman, A.L., *The Fat Flush Plan.* 2002, New York: McGraw-Hill.

Gittleman, A.L. and J.M. Desgrey, *Beyond Pritikin.* 1988, New York: Bantam Books.

Guyton, A.C., *Textbook of Medical Physiology.* 1986, Philadelphia: W.B. Saunders Company. 438-450, 876-966.

Haller, C.A. and N.L. Benowitz, "Adverse Cardiovascular and Central Nervous System Events Associated with Dietary Supplements Containing Ephedra Alkaloids." *Massachusetts Medical Society*, 2000.

Hamadeh, M.J. and et. al., "Nutritional Aspects of Flaxseed in the Human Diet". *Proceedings of the Flaxseed Institute*, 1992. 4: 48-53.

Hart, C., *Secrets of Serotonin.* 1996, New York: Lynn Sonberg Book Associates.

Hawkins, D.R., M.D., Ph.D., *Power Vs. Force.* 5 ed. 1995, Sedona: Veritas Publishing.

Heleniak, E.P. and B. Aston, *Prostaglandins, Brown Fat, and Weight Loss.* Medical Hypothesis, 1989. 28: 13-33.

Hibbeln, J.R. and N. Salem, "Dietary polyunsaturated fatty acids and depression: when cholesterol does not satisfy." *American Journal of Clinical Nutrition*, July 1995. 62: 1-9.

Hirohata, T., et. al., "An Epidemiologic Study on the Association Between Diet and Breast Cancer." *Journal of the National Cancer Institute*, 1987. 78(1): 595-600.

Hoffman, D.M. and et. al., "Diagnosis of Growth Hormone Deficiency in Adults." *Lancet*, 1994. 343: 1064-1068.

Hogan, E.H., B.A. Hornick, and A. Bouchoux, "Communicating the Message: Clarifying the Controversies about Caffeine" *Nutrition Today*. Jan/Feb 2002. 28-35.

Horrocks, L.A. and Y.K. Yeo, "Health Benefits of Docosahexaenoic (DHA)." *Pharmacological Research*, 1999. 40(3): 211-225.

Hu, F.B. and et. al., "A Prospective Study of Egg Consumption and Risk of Cardiovascular Disease in Men and Women." *Journal of the American Medical Association*, 1999. 281: 1387-94.

Hudson, T., "The Good Fat for Women." *Health Products Business*. 2000. 25-26.

Janda, J., "The War on Obesity." *Club Industry*. Jan 2000. 10-14.

Jenkins, D.J.A., et. al., "Glycemic Index of Foods: A Physiological Basis for Carbohydrate Exchange." *American Journal of Clinical Nutrition*, 1981. 34: 363-66.

Kaplan, P., "But What Should I Eat?" *Personal Fitness Professional*. 2002. 18-21.

Kaplan, P., "The Diet Roller Coaster Ride." *Personal Fitness Professional*. March 2002. 26-30.

Keys, A., *Seven Countries: A Multivariate Analysis of Death and Coronary Heart Disease*. 1980, Cambridge: Harvard University Press.

Kirschenbauer, H.G., *Fats and Oils: An Outline of their Chemistry and Technology*. 2 ed. 1960, New York: Van Nostrand Reinhold.

Klatz, R., *Grow Young with HGH*. 1997, New York: Harper-Collins.

Kraemer, W.J., "Influence of the endocrine system on resistance training adaptations." *National Strength & Conditioning Association Journal*, 1992. 14: 47-53.

Leahy, M., R. Roderick, and K. Brillian, "The Cranberry-Promising Health Benefits, Old and New." *Nutrition Today*. Sep/Oct 2001. 241-248.

Leitzmann, M.F. and et. al., "Prospective Study of Coffee Consumption and the Risk of Symptomatic Gallstones in Men." *Journal of the American Medical Association*, 1999. 281: 2106-12.

Ludwig, D.S. and et. al., "High Glycemic Index Foods, Overeating and Obesity." *Pediatrics*, 1999. 103: 61-66.

Mather, A., "All about antioxidants." *Vegetarian Times*. Dec 2000. 73-74.

McBean, L.D., et al., "Healthy Eating in Later Years." *Nutrition Today*. July/Aug 2001. 192-201.

McCarthy, D., "Long-Chain Omega-3 Fatty Acids and Cardiovascular Health." *Scan's Pulse*. 2002. 1-3.

Mensink, R.P. and M.B. Katan, "Effect of Dietary Trans Fatty Acids on High-density and Low-density Lipoprotein Cholesterol Level in Healthy Subjects." *New England Journal of Medicine*, 1990. 323: 439-45.

Messina, M. and S. Barnes, "The Role of Soy Products in Reducing Risk of Cancer." *Journal of the National Cancer Institute*, 1991. 83(8): 541-546.

Mindell, E., R.Ph., Ph.D, *Earl Mindell's Soy Miracle*. 1995, New York.

Morris, D.H., "Essential Nutrients and Other Functional Compounds in Flaxseed." *Nutrition Today*. 2001. 159-162.

Murray, M.T. and J. Beutler, *Understanding Fats and Oils*. 1996, Encinitas: Progressive Health Publishing.

Myers, R.L., *NutraSweet: Friend or Foe?* Health Consultants Limited.

Nachtigall, L., *Estrogen: The Facts Can Change Your Life*. 1994, New York: Harper & Collins.

Null, G., *Gary Null's Ultimate Lifetime Diet*. Broadway Publishing.

Ornish, D., *Dr. Dean Ornish's Program for Reversing Heart Disease*. 1990, New York: Random House.

Ornish, D., *Eat More, Weigh Less*. 1993, New York: Harper Collins.

Page, L., *Healthy Healing: an alternative healing reference*. 8 ed. 1990, San Francisco: Author Published.

Papas, P.N., C.A. Brusch, and G.C. Ceresia, *Cranberry Juice in the Treatment of Urinary Tract Infections*. Southwest Med, 1966. 47: 17-20.

Peek, W.A. and et. al., "Research Directions in Osteoporosis." *American Journal of Medicine*, 1988. 84: 275-282.

Peeke, P., *Fight Fat after Forty*. 2000, New York: Penguin.

Perkins, E.C. and W.J. Visek, "Dietary Fats and Health." *American Oil Chemists' Society*. 1983: Champaign.

Peterson, G. and S. Barnes, "Genistein Inhibition of the Growth of Human Breast Cancer Cells: Independence from Estrogen Receptors and the Multi-Drug Resistance Chain." *Biochemical and Biophysical Research Communications*, 1991. 179(1): 661-667.

Peterson, G. and S. Barnes, "Genistein and Biochanan A Inhibit the Growth of Human Prostate Cancer Cells but Not Epidermal Growth Factor Receptor Tyrosine Autophosphorylation." *The Prostate*, 1993. 22: 335-345.

Rabat, M., "The Great Pyramid." *Vegetarian Times*. 2001. 12.

Richard, D., *Stevia Rebaudiana: Nature's Sweet Secret.* 3 ed. 1999, Bloomingdale: Vital Health Publishing.

Rudin, D., M.D. and C. Felix, *Omega-3 Oils; A Practical Guide.* 1996, Garden City: Avery Publishing Group. 1-24, 39-49.

Rudin, D., M.D., C. Felix, and C. Schrader, *The Omega-3 Phenomenon: The Nutritional Breakthrough of the 80's.* 1987, New York: Rawson Associates.

Schmid, R.E., "Government moves to require trans fat listing on food labels." *Lansing State Journal*. 2002: Lansing. 6A.

Schwartz, R., *Diets Don't Work.* 1982, Houston: Breakthru Publishing.

Sears, B., Ph.D., *Enter The Zone.* 1 ed. 1995, New York: Harper & Collins.

Sears, B., Ph.D., *The Anti-Aging Zone.* 1999, New York: Harper & Collins.

Selye, H., *Stress Without Distress.* 1974, New York: Harper & Row.

Simopoulos, A.P., "Omega-3 Fatty Acids in Health and Chronic Disease and in Growth and Development." *American Journal of Clinical Nutrition*, 1991. 54: 438-463.

Simopoulos, A.P., ed. "Metabolic Consequences of Changing Dietary Patterns." *World Review of Nutrition and Dietetics*, 1996. 79.

Simopoulos, A.P., "Essential Fatty Acids in Health and Chronic Disease." *American Journal of Clinical Nutrition*, 1999. 70: 560s-569s.

Simopoulos, A.P. and J. Robinson, *The Omega Plan*. 1 ed, New York: Harper Collins.

Slavin, J., "Nutritional Benefits of Soy Protein and Soy Fiber." *Journal of the American Dietetic Association*, 1991. 91: 816-819.

Smith, L.H., *Improving Your Child's Behavior Chemistry*. 1984, Englewood Cliffs: Prentice-Hall.

Snyder, D.K. and et. al., "Anabolic Effects of Growth Hormone in Obese Diet Restricted Subjects are Dose Dependent." *American Journal of Clinical Nutrition*, 1990. 52: 431-437.

Spagnoli, A. and et. al., "Long-term acetyl-l-carnitine treatment in Alzheimer's disease." *Neurology*, 1991. 41: 1726-1732.

Spruce, N. and A. Titchenal, *An Evaluation of Popular Fitness-Enhancing Supplements*. 2001: Evergreen Communications.

Stein, J., "The Low-Carb Diet Craze." *Time*. Nov 1999. 72-79.

Stevens, L.J. and et. al., "Omega-3 Fatty Acids in Boys with Behavior, Learning, and Health Problems." *Physiology and Behavior*, 1996. 59(4-5): 915-920.

Taubes, G., "The Soft Science of Dietary Fat." *Science*. 2001. 2536-2545.

Tillotson, J.E., "Our Ready-Prepared Ready-to-Eat Nation." *Nutrition Today*. Jan/Feb 2002. 36-38.

U.S.D.A. Services, "Food Guide Pyramid." *National Cattleman's Beef Association*. 1993.

Washburn, S. and et. al., "Effect of Soy Protein Supplementation on Serum Lipoproteins, Blood Pressure, and Menopausal Symptoms in Perimenopausal Women." *Menopause*, 1999. 6: 7-13.

Weiss, R., "A Shot at Youth." *Health*. 1993. 38-47.

Wheeler, G.D. and et. al.,
"Endurance Training
Decreases Testosterone Levels
in Men without Change in
Luteinizing Hormone."
*Journal of Clinical
Endocrinological Metabolism*,
1991. 42: 422-425.

Willett, W.C., *Eat, Drink, and
Be Healthy.* 2001, New York:
Simon & Schuster.

Willett, W.C. and et. al.,
"Mediterranean Diet Pyramid:
A Cultural Model for Healthy
Eating." *American Journal
of Clinical Nutrition*, 1995.
61: S1402-6.

Williams, K.V. and M.T.
Korytkowski, "Syndrome X:
Pathogenesis, Clinical and
Therapeutic Aspects."
*Diabetes Nutrition and
Metabolism*, 1998. 11: 140-152.

Yehl, T., *Perfect Form Strength
Training*, East Lansing:
Myotech Health & Fitness Inc.

Young, V.R., "Good Nutrition
for All: Challenge for the
Nutritional Sciences in the
New Millennium." *Nutrition
Today.* Jan/Feb 2001.

Index